A Workbook on Human Spermatozoa and Assisted Conception

A Workbook on Human Spermatozoa and Assisted Conception

Editors

Sonia Malik DGO MD FICOG FIAMS
Programme Director
Southend Fertility and IVF Centre
Holy Angels Hospital
Vasant Vihar, New Delhi, India

Ashok Agarwal PhD HCLD (ABB) EMB (ACE)
Director
Center for Reproductive Medicine
Professor
Case Western Reserve University and
Lerner College of Medicine
Cleveland Clinic
Cleveland, Ohio 44195, USA

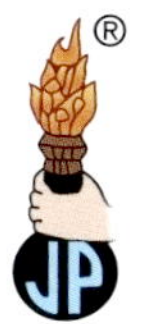

JAYPEE BROTHERS MEDICAL PUBLISHERS (P) LTD

New Delhi • Panama City • London

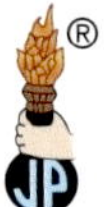

Jaypee Brothers Medical Publishers (P) Ltd.

Headquarter

Jaypee Brothers Medical Publishers (P) Ltd
4838/24, Ansari Road, Daryaganj
New Delhi 110 002, India
Phone: +91-11-43574357
Fax: +91-11-43574314
Email: jaypee@jaypeebrothers.com

Overseas Offices

J.P. Medical Ltd.,
83 Victoria Street London
SW1H 0HW (UK)
Phone: +44-2031708910
Fax: +02-03-0086180
Email: info@jpmedpub.com

Jaypee-Highlights Medical Publishers Inc.
City of Knowledge, Bld. 237, Clayton
Panama City, Panama
Phone: 507-317-0160
Fax: +50-73-010499
Email: cservice@jphmedical.com

Website: www.jaypeebrothers.com
Website: www.jaypeedigital.com

Inquiries for bulk sales may be solicited at: jaypee@jaypeebrothers.com

Publisher: Jitendar P Vij
Publishing Director: Tarun Duneja
Cover Design: Seema Dogra

A Workbook on Human Spermatozoa and Assisted Conception

First Edition: **2012**

ISBN 978-93-5025-517-9

Printed at Replika Press Pvt. Ltd.

Contributors

Alex C Verghese PhD
Scientific Director
Albany Molecular Research Inc. (AMRI)—
in vitro Fertilization (IVF)
Kolkata, West Bengal, India

Ashok Agarwal PhD HCLD (ABB) EMB (ACE)
Director
Center for Reproductive Medicine
Professor
Case Western Reserve University and
Lerner College of Medicine, Cleveland Clinic
Cleveland, Ohio 44195, USA

Juan G Alvarez MD PhD
Centro ANDROGEN
La Caruna, Spain

Kuldeep Jain MD
Fellow
Assisted Reproductive Technology (ART)
(Singapore)
Director, KJIVF and Laparoscopy Centre
Delhi, India

Lt Col Pankaj Talwar VSM
Head of the Department
Assisted Reproductive Technology (ART)
Centre
Army Hospital (Research and Referral)
New Delhi, India

MM Misro PhD Post Doc (USA)
Professor
Department of Reproductive Biomedicine
National Health Family Welfare Institution
(NHFWI), Munirka, New Delhi, India

Rima Dada MD PhD
Laboratory for Molecular Reproduction
and Genetics
Department of Anatomy
All India Institute of Medical Sciences
(AIIMS)
New Delhi, India

RK Sharma VSM
Head of Department
Assisted Reproductive Technology (ART)
Centre
Armed Forces Medical College (AFMC)
Pune, Maharashtra, India

Sandro C Esteves MD PhD
Andrology and Human Reproduction Clinic
(ANDROFERT)
Campinas, Brazil

Savita Nagpal MD (Path)
Director
Dr Savita Nagpal's Pathlab
Vasant Kunj
New Delhi, India

Shubhangi Gangal PhD
Uma Fertility and IVF Centre
Thane, Maharashtra, India

Ved Prakash BSc BAMS
Southend Fertility and IVF Centre
Holy Angels Hospital
Vasant Vihar
New Delhi, India

Prologue

The sperm was discovered many centuries ago—much before man got the first glimpse of the oocyte, yet male infertility remains an enigma today. Even advances like intracytoplasmic sperm injection (ICSI) in the management of male infertility have not been able to increase pregnancy rates. This is because very little attention has been paid to this cause of infertility. The last decade has, however, seen an explosion in research in this area. Some clouds are parting but a lot needs to be done before we can see bright sunshine.

Southend Fertility and *in vitro* fertilization (IVF) centre, New Delhi, India, has been striving for academic excellence ever since its inception in 2001. Our practice in all these years helped us to recognize these gaps in the treatment of the male. It was this need that drove us to organize this workshop and symposium.

Reactive oxygen species (ROS) and deoxyribonucleic acid (DNA) damage lead to unhealthy sperms which may not lead to a pregnancy. It is, therefore, important to look more closely at the sperm function and morphology. New advances in this field are the highlights of this workshop. Intricate details of intracytoplasmic sperm injection (ICSI) are found in the chapter on micromanipulation but even that is now said to be incomplete without selection of the morphologically normal sperm or intracytoplasmic morphologically-selected sperm injection (IMSI), a new advance in ART that needs to be mastered by all practicing ICSI.

Exemplary work in this field has been done by Dr Ashok Agarwal and his team at Cleveland Clinic. It is our great fortune and good luck that we have been able to organize this workshop with him, Prof Juan G Alvarez and Dr Sandro C Esteves, all stalwarts in andrology. We are also fortunate to have an equally reputed national faculty.

As an introduction to the subject, the first few chapters in the workbook describe the equipment and media, simplified protocols for semen analysis, semen preparation in various situations. A lucid description of semen banking can be found in the workbook since it forms an integral part of any assisted reproductive technology (ART) unit.

We thank our faculty for demonstrating in this extraordinary workshop that describes not only the basic structure and function of the sperm but also its use in intricate procedures like IMSI and ICSI.

The workshop is an attempt to present evidence-based procedures and practices that are presently evolving or are being carried out on the human spermatozoa in ART. This workbook is a compilation of what is being demonstrated in the workshop. We hope this will be a useful tool for all practicing ART.

Sonia Malik DGO MD FICOG FIAMS

Aug. 2011
New Delhi

Contents

Introduction

The field of human-assisted reproduction is growing by leaps and bounds with recent advances in areas of embryo culture, vitrification, Preimplantation genetic diagnosis (PGD), new WHO guidelines for semen examination and the latest techniques for the surgical retrieval and methods for the selection of best spermatozoa. However, the advances in this promising field are being severely threatened due to the lack of rigorous training and availability of laboratory personnel qualified to work in the human embryology clinics in less developed or in more developed countries.

I am pleased that the hands on training workshop on *Human Spermatozoa and Assisted Conception* being organized on 12th August, 2011 at the India Habitat Center, New Delhi, India, is a bold attempt to empower reproductive professionals interested in in-depth training and knowledge of some of the most important techniques and protocols related to andrology and embryology.

The information compiled in this workbook is taken from both international and Indian experts engaged in assisted reproductive procedures. The 17 chapters included in this book contain practical information, step by step protocols, list of supplies and equipment and selected references.

I am confident that manual will be of immediate help to all those interested in the field of assisted reproductive technologies (ARTs). The readers can learn and master various sophisticated techniques included in this manual and in turn contribute to improvements in ART outcome of individual clinics.

Sincerely,

Ashok Agarwal PhD HCLD (ABB) EMB (ACE)
Director, Center for Reproductive Medicine
Professor, Case Western Reserve University and
Lerner College of Medicine
Cleveland Clinic
Cleveland, Ohio 44195, USA

1 Equipment and Culture Media

RK Sharma

INTRODUCTION

A well-planned laboratory is the foundation of a successful *in vitro* fertilization (IVF) practice. There are several factors that should be taken into consideration when designing the laboratory. The equipment you choose is as important as the laboratory space itself. The success of an IVF lab is dependent on the conditions in the laboratory. The media you use should be conducive to the environment and the working culture of the laboratory.

Workstations need to be positioned sensibly and logically to make working more practical and accident free. Efficiency and safety should be considered when positioning incubators, centrifuges, flow cabinets and cryopreservation equipment.

In addition, local health and safety guidelines must be complied with. A sterile environment should be maintained in the laboratory with rigorous daily cleaning of floors and surfaces. This is of particular importance in areas where tissue culture techniques are applied, such as media making, to prevent any microbial contamination. If the andrology and embryology areas are within a single setting, it is advisable to allocate separate incubators for each to prevent temperature and pH fluctuations every time the incubator door is opened.

The IVF laboratory should be located in a low traffic area and entry restrictions should apply. Careful attention has to be paid to the type of paint used as the use of solvent-based paints is lethal to embryos. Low fume or water-based paint should be used on the walls and surrounding area. It is recommended that the paintwork should be completed at least two weeks before starting laboratory work involving oocytes and embryos. The use of strong adhesives also should be avoided for the same reasons.

It is best to have vinyl or single-layered flooring which is antistatic. Wooden or tiled floors should be avoided as their crevices and ridges can trap dirt and they are more difficult to clean. The benches should be of an adequate height to enable comfortable working. Adjustable height chairs are quite useful. These should be PVC or leather-coated to avoid the accumulation of dust in fabric covers.

The laboratory should ideally be located next to the theater where oocyte recovery and embryo transfers are carried out. The size of the laboratory depends on several factors, such as the number of embryologists, the equipment, the number of cycles performed and whether specialized treatments are performed (such as preimplantation genetic diagnosis on sperm washing for HIV positive patients). The laboratory should have an adequate space to ensure aseptic and optimal handling of the gametes and the embryos at all times.

EQUIPMENT

- Incubators
- Isolates
- IVF workstation
- Stereo zoom microscope
- Aspiration pump
- Laminar flow
- Ambient filter system
- Test tube warmers
- Heater plates
- Slow freezing devices
- Makler counting chambers
- Phase contrast microscope
- Centrifuge
- Refrigerators
- Micromanipulators with inverted microscope
- Laser system
- Automatic sperm analyzers
- Sperm class analyzer
- Antivibration platform and table.

Incubators

These are virtual fallopian tubes and high performing incubators are critical for the success of an IVF lab. Reliability and consistency are absolutely necessary.

The incubator can be water jacketed or air jacketed. Water jacketed incubators have a large thermal mass, so do not cool down as much when opening the door and during power failures. Air-jacketed technology is lightweighted and is of low maintenance. Therefore, such technology provides additional protection of high temperature contamination control. Air-jacketed incubators are preferred for better decontamination function.

The inner chambers of incubators may have a steel, copper or copper enriched steel inner sheet. CO_2 incubators with copper in their cabinet are designed to deter contamination. As the copper breaks down, it releases copper oxide, which destroys microbes present in the chamber. The microbiocidal action is only when copper comes in contact with water, however, they are difficult to maintain and require frequent cleaning. Unless new particles are exposed by some sort of metal removal process like sanding down the inner chamber, the antimicrobial benefits would slowly disappear. For low maintenance and easy cleaning, steel lined cabinets are preferred.

Incubation of live cells requires precise control of environmental parameters such as temperature, humidity and pH. Carbon dioxide lowers the pH in the chamber of an incubator to levels similar to that of the natural mammalian body environment and is a critical element in incubation. The sensors for controlling CO_2 are based on Thermal conductivity (TC) or Infrared (IR) technology. TC sensors provide accurate CO_2 control in applications where temperature and humidity values are consistent. IR sensors are recommended in uses where temperature and humidity are changed frequently. Further the IR sensors can be single or dual, of them the latter is better. These sensors could have remote alarm contacts by SIM message or connection to inhouse alarm system.

The door of incubators is equally important for maintaining humidity, temperature and pH. Instead of single door, multiple door screen is beneficial for culturing oocytes and embryos as this will minimize the rate of CO_2 loss and rapid drops in temperature when the door is opened. The six door model is preferred over others for better temperature and CO_2 control.

The incubators are needed to maintain humidity by incorporating water trays. Nowadays unique panless humidity system is available which generates relatively high humidity protecting cultures and prevents them from drying out. Humidity recovery times are up to five times faster than those of standard water tray. Humidity poses the risk of fungal and bacterial contamination. Some incubators come with a built-in 'disinfection routine' module which is useful for cleaning (the walls and plates heat up to 90°C) aka CONTRACAN. These cycles could be moist heat cycle of 90°C or moist plus dry heat. The Galaxy incubators from RS Biotech have a high-heat decon feature, which the Hera-cell line also has. The decon feature is nice, as it heats up the incubator to 200 degrees to kill any germs.

Incubators may have internal fan to circulate the gas and heat. Incubator that does not have a fan or other moving parts reduces contamination and particle production. But these incubators have some problems in maintaining pH.

Another vital consideration is to have a CO_2 or TRI Gas incubators. For blastocyst culture, low oxygen is required. Current literature suggests the use of 5% O_2 for extended culture However, studies with mouse ova have shown spindle damage and unaligned chromosomes in low oxygen tensions (Hu et al. 2001). Some incubators have got HEPA filter for inner circulating air. These filters need to be changed every six months.

Incubators should be cleaned at least once a month with 70% ethanol (analar grade) and flushed out with one liter of sterile water (tissue culture grade non-pyrogenic). They should be left running overnight after cleaning before culturing gametes or embryos.

Benchtop Incubators

These are the new generation incubators and are compact with a very small chamber volume. They can easily fit over the workstation. They reduce transit time between the incubator and the workstation, besides low gas consumption.

Their main advantage is the rapid recovery of CO_2 and temperature within three minutes of opening the chamber lid. It does this by purging the gas at a rate of 25 mL/min in the chamber. It uses a tri gas mixture of 5% O_2, 6% CO_2 and 89% nitrogen, which is quite expensive compared to pure clinical grade CO_2. They can be used for conventional IVF.

Temperature recovery after a 5-s door opening/closing procedure is approximately 5 minutes for the mini-incubator and 30 minutes for the conventional incubator. The oxygen concentration return is significantly improved in the mini-incubator (3.0 +/–0 min) compared with the conventional incubator (7.8 +/–0.9 min). Both the early-stage good embryo formation rate and the good blastocyst formation rate are significantly higher in the mini-incubator (39.5% and 15.1%) than the conventional incubator (28.4% and 7.8%). The microenvironment maintenance ability of incubators appears to significantly influence the formation of good embryos (Fujiwara et al. 2007).

The benchtop incubator is much easier to clean than the conventional one. It uses 150 mL of water as opposed to 5 l with the conventional one. However, they can only contain a maximum of eight dishes which means that bigger laboratories may need three to four incubators.

Benchtop incubators have to be installed with autodiallers that will dial out in cases of incubator emergencies. In case of a power cut or CO_2 depletion, the chamber will maintain its pH and temperature for about an hour if unopened which gives the embryologist some time to rectify the problem. Incubators should also have two tanks of CO_2/mixed gas attached to a changeover unit, in case one runs out so that the other is activated immediately. All fittings and silcone tubing should be checked for leaks. Incubators should be fully serviced twice yearly.

MINC or BT37 both are capable of supporting embryo growth with reduced oxygen levels and both have broadly similar features. BT37 takes care of issues of cranked and water clogged humidity tubing by employing tube guides and heaters. It also comes with built-in battery power which lasts for two hours. There is also a visual indication for active humidification. The heating plate(s) are calibrated at six different points as against other incubators.

Laminar Flow

The laminar flow hood provides an aseptic work area while allowing the containment of infectious splashes or aerosols generated by many microbiological procedures. Three kinds of laminar flow hoods, designated as Classes I, II and III, have been developed to meet varying research and clinical needs.

Class I laminar flow hoods offer significant levels of protection to laboratory personnel and to the environment when used with various microbiological techniques but they do not provide cultures protection from contamination. They are similar in design and air flow characteristics to chemical fume hoods.

Class II laminar flow hoods are designed for work involving BSL-1, 2 and 3 materials, and they also provide an aseptic environment necessary for cell culture experiments. A Class II biosafety cabinet should be used for handling potentially hazardous materials (e.g. primate-derived cultures, virally infected cultures, radioisotopes, carcinogenic or toxic reagents).

Class III biosafety cabinets are gas-tight and they provide the highest attainable level of protection to personnel and the environment. A Class III biosafety cabinet is required for work involving known human pathogens and other BSL-4 material.

Laminar flow hoods protect the working enviroment from dust and other airborn contaminants by maintaining a constant, unidirectional flow of HEPA-filtered air over the work area. The flow can be horizontal, blowing parallel to the work surface, or it can be vertical, blowing from the top of the cabinet onto the work surface.

Depending on its design, a horizontal flow hood provides protection to the culture (if the air flowing towards the user) or to the user (if the air is drawn in through the front of the cabinet by negative air pressure inside). Vertical flow hoods, on the other hand, provide significant protection to the user and the cell culture.

Clean Benches

Horizontal laminar flow or vertical laminar flow "clean benches" are not biosafety cabinets; these pieces of equipment discharge HEPA-filtered air from the back of the cabinet across the work surface toward the user, and they may expose the user to potentially hazardous materials. These devices only provide product protection. Clean benches can be used for certain clean activities, such as the dust-free assembly of sterile equipment or electronic devices, and they should never be used when handling cell culture materials or drug formulations, or when manipulating potentially infectious materials. Recent guidelines suggest that vertical flow cabinets should be used to handle samples from patients with HIV or hepatitis B or C. They should be kept clean at all times and the number of items inside the flow hood should be minimized to ensure that the air flow is not disrupted. The flow cabinets should be serviced annually with filter changes every six months.

Culture Lab Air Cleaner (Coda Air Filtration System)

Awareness about air quality has increased in the last few years. Air contaminants include: volatile organic compounds (VOCs) such as aldehydes; small organic molecules such as nitric oxide, sulphur dioxide and carbon monoxide (from exhaust fumes); and liquids such as floor wax that contains heavy metals. The degree of pollution depends on the location of the IVF unit. Urban laboratories are more likely to have higher pollution. Contaminants in the ambient air will also circulate through the incubators. Cohen et al. (1997) showed that certain adhesives arrested >90% of mouse embryos at the 2-cell stage with very low blastocyst formation. Brand new incubators emit>100 times higher concentrations of VOCs than used ones (Cohen et al. 1997). Many laboratories have a positive pressure HEPA filtration system to extract inorganic contaminants (e.g. dust, bacteria). Additional absorption systems containing activated carbon and potassium permanganate are required to remove VOCs. Airconditioning systems should recirculate HEPAa-filtered air rather than draw air from the outside.

The incubator filter contains activated carbon and conveniently fits into an incubator compartment. It purifies the air by reducing VOCs, heavy metals and chemical air contaminants. The filters are changed monthly or every time the incubators are cleaned.

The filtration towers incorporate a four-stage filter, which contains a unique blend of activated carbon, alumina impregnated with potassium permanganate for absorption and oxidation of a wide variety of gases and particulate contaminants. It removes up to 99% of all contaminants by filtration through 0.2 µm filters and performs 12 to 15 air exchanges per hour. The number of Coda Towers needed depends on the size of the laboratory (one tower for 300 square feet).

The filters are changed quarterly with a yearly general service. In line CO_2 filters are installed in the tubing between the CO_2 tanks and the incubator. This filter is suitable for tri-gas as well as pure CO_2. These filters can also be attached to CO_2 controlled environmental chambers used for routine embryology.

GenX Coda Aero towers, ZANDAIR and *zIVF-AIRe and many more are available, they are equally good or bad and require periodic check for VOC and the HEPA filters.*

In Vitro Fertilization (IVF) Workstation

This is a controlled environmental chamber which is mobile and is specifically designed to maintain ideal temperature and pH during the handling of gametes and embryos. The working chamber is maintained at a temperature of 37°C with 5 to 6% CO_2 in air. Temperature is monitored by a thermostat and CO_2 levels by an infrared sensor. A dissecting microscope is needed for egg collections inseminations, fertilization checks, denuding eggs for ICSI (intracytoplasmic sperm injection), normal evaluation and grading of embryos and embryo transfers.

Several studies have shown that prolonged temperature fluctuations can be very detrimental to the meiotic spindle in human oocytes. This can lead to chromosomal aberrations in the resulting embryo with a reduced chance of implantation. The IVF chamber is ideal for training embryologists as temperature fluctuations are minimized if the manipulation takes longer than expected.

Heated stages for oocytes and embryo viewing are necessary. Prolonged exposure of oocytes and embryos to temperatures below 37°C can disrupt their cytoskeleton. All microscopes used for gametes and embryos should have heated stages. Heated stages can be installed on most brands of dissecting microscopes (Nikon, Hunter Scientific). A heated surface with a wide working area can also be incorporated in a Class II flow cabinet.

It is suggested that the stage temperature is set slightly higher than 37°C so that the drops of media with the embryos or oocytes are maintained at 37°C. It is advisable to experiment with a dish without embryos (in the system that you intend to use) to determine the ideal temperature setting.

Microscopes

Good microscopes are required for routine embryological and andrological procedures. A dissecting microscope is essential to score oocyte cumulii complex, pronuclei and embryos for transfer. The range of its magnification should be between 20 and 160x.

A phase contrast microscope is needed to score detailed semen parameters such as morphology. Some clinics use the computer aided semen analysis system (CASA) to reduce interobserver variation.

Micromanipulation

A micromanipulator is necessary for ICSI and embryo biopsy for preimplantation genetic diagnosis. In addition, a good inverted microscope with a heated stage and a magnification of up to 400x is needed. The controls can be either pneumatic or hydraulic. Although hydraulic syringes have more effective control and movement, they can be fairly time-consuming and messy to prime the tubing with oil every time there is trapped air within the system. The micromanipulation system should be placed in a vibration-free environment. Hydraulically controlled antivibration tables are commercially available. If there is limited air filtration in the laboratory, the micromanipulator system can be placed within a class II flow hood. When choosing the manipulators, it is very important to consider the ease of manoeuvrability.

Some systems have automated and complicated electrical controls whereas some are more manual. The simpler the system, the easier it is to rectify problems in an emergency without the need to call in a technician. For units performing embryo biopsy, a triple tool holder may be necessary to breach the zona. However, if an infrared laser system is installed then a dual tool holder should be sufficient to perform he procedure. For teaching purposes, it is advisable to have a video-linked camera mounted on the micromanipulator. This is also useful to record embryo biopsies and look back to detect any contamination of cumulus cells. A commonly used micromanipulator systems are Research Instruments, Narashige, and Eppendorf.

Disposable micropipettes are available commercially from Cook, Humagen, RI etc. The Integra Ti™ by Research Instruments is currently leader in pack. It is accurate, simple to use and reliable. It has been designed to offer the ultimate in user control. Simple pipette set-up and angle adjustment reduce the time of ICSI procedures, therefore optimizing the results.

Ovum Aspiration Pump

It creates a negative pressure and is used for ovum pickups. It has foot operated switch with vacuum gauze variable from 0 to 500 mm Hg. Fluid trap prevents aspiration of fluid into vacuum unit.

Rocket Pumps are reliable and available many years ago, Cook has come with new pump. Both are equally good.

Controlled Rate Freezing System/Cryosystems

CryoMed Freezers for IVF are designed for human *in vitro* fertilization with precise control, ease of setup and operation, and convenience. Chamber, sample temperature and operation status are continuously displayed on the control panel. These IVF models provide convenient front and top access for easy sample "seeding".

They are hardly used with vetrification in vogue nowadays. While different cryosystems are available having different instruments, we are using open system McGill Cryoleaf by Origio.

General Equipment

Centrifuge

Centrifuge is used for density gradient semen preparation. Nowadays good centrifuges are available which can be programmed to give accurate g force. REMI centrifuges are used by our lab.

Refrigerator/Freezer

It is used to store culture media and other media used for embryology and andrology. Culture media are very temperature sensitive. Certain amino acids and proteins in the media can be inactivated by extreme temperatures and hence should be kept at 2 to 8°C.

Dry Heat Oven for Sterilizing

It is used for drying and sterilizing glass pipettes and other nondisposable items such as tweezers, spatulas and media-making glassware.

A pH meter and an osmometer are designed for particular laboratories making their own media.

All laboratory equipment should be easy to use and to maintain, besides having good service and repair facility. A log of servicing and maintenance should be kept.

Makler's Chamber/Phase Contrast Microscope

These are inescapable requirement for andrology lab and you should go for the best available. Indian equipment is equally good and we have used them for package.

Laser-Assisted System for PGD and Hatching

Saturn 3 by RI or XY Clone by Hamilton Throne are available and can be integrated into the ICSI micromanipulator. The software and accuracy of Saturn system is slightly better than that of Hamilton.

Labware and Disposables

All plasticware that is used in the laboratory should be proven to be nonembryotoxic. The most commonly used plasticware in IVF laboratories are supplied by equipment companies. All the plastic ware should be disposable and not re-used under any circumstances. All new batches should undergo in-house quality control testing before use. Batches that fail in-house checks should be returned. If possible, new packs of dishes should be opened for each patient or each working day to keep the contents sterile. Resealing opened packs should be kept to a minimum. It is strongly recommended to use individually wrapped sterile pipette tips and plastic pipettes for inseminations and sperm preparation. This will minimize the potential risk of any cross-contamination.

Glass pipettes used for routine embryology should be borosilicate and not the cheaper soda glass since these are thought to leach minerals into the culture media. The pipettes should be double washed in sterile water before being plugged with cotton wool and sterilized at 100°C. Glass pipettes should be stored in special metal canisters and the number of pipettes in each should be kept to a minimum so that a new sterile can is opened each day. All pipettes should be flame polished before use. Presterilized (gamma irradiated) and plugged pipettes are also commercially available.

Sterile nontoxic powder-free latex gloves should be worn during embryo transfer. The powder can be embryotoxic if it enters the dish. Gloves minimize the introduction of contaminants and skin flora, into the incubator or culture system.

Ovum Pickup Needles

Ovum pickup needle is used for ovum aspiration with help of TV probe and aspiration pump. It is designed for precise recovery with minimal trauma. It is available with single and double lumen systems with a choice of 16G or 17G SS needle. Ecomarking maximizes ultrasound visibility.

We generally use Wallace or Cooks single lumen pickup needles.

Embryo Transfer Catheter

This catheter is used for transvaginal transfer of embryos into uterus along with tissue culture medium with ultrasound guided marking and available in different sizes. Being designed to avoid embryo damage, the inner catheter is made of medical grade polyurethane which is known to be non embryotoxic. The hand finished round tip prevents traumatic introduction and graduation on the inner catheter allows alignment with the outer sheath, producing a smooth radius for minimal trauma during insertion.

The choice of embryo transfer catheter is a joint decision between the clinician and the embryologist. Several factors have be taken into account when deciding which catheter to use. These are:

- The material used in making the catheter (embryo safe)
- Packaging/sterility
- The lumen diameter of the inner sheath and the ease of loading the embryos
- Embryos should be released in a minimum amount of medium
- The ease of cannulating the cervix
- Cost
- Any clinical trial result.

Oocyte Preparation Pipettes

It is used for the transfer of the oocyte or embryos from dish to dish. The tip is well rounded by fire polishing. Available in different IDs as per application.

Denudation Pipettes

It is used for the denudation of the oocyte before the microinjection by ICSI. Cumulus mass and corona tissues are removed by repeated aspiration and expiration of the oocyte. Available in different ID as per application.

Holding Pipettes

Used for ICSI, assisted hatching and blastomere biopsy. The well shaped fire polished tip allows secure fixation of oocyte and avoids damage of cell. Maximal contact surface, 95 micron or 120 micron OD, bend angle available from 5 to 35 degree.

Injection Pipette

Used to perform intracytoplasmic sperm injection into oocytes. It is available with/without heat formed spike having different angles, spiked or hypodermic bevel. Four to six micron ID, bend angles available 5 to 35 degree.

Apart from the above the labware used is as under

- Conical tube 15 mL (Falcon ref. 3215/3217)
- Centrifuge tube 4 mL (Falcon ref. 2003)
- Plate with center well 60 mm (Falcon ref. 3037)
- Plate without center well 60 mm (Falcon ref. 3002)
- Plate 35 mm (Falcon ref. 3001)
- Plate 50 mm (Falcon ref. 1006)
- Transfer pipette 3 mL (Falcon ref. 7575)
- Pipette 10 mL (Falcon ref. 7551)
- Pipette 5 mL (Falcon ref. 7543)
- Flask 50 mL (Falcon ref. 3013)
- Flask 200 mL (Falcon ref. 3024)
- 4 well plates (Nunc ref. 176740)
- Glass mark pen (ref. 750 – Glass mark pen)
- Stripper (MID Atlantic Diagnosis Inc.)
- Stripper Tips 200 μm (ref. MXL3-200); 150 μm (ref. MXLE-150); 125 μm (ref. MXL3-125).

CULTURE MEDIA FOR IVF

Culture media for embryo development must meet the metabolic needs of preimplantation embryos by addressing amino acid and energy requirements based on the specific developmental stage of the embryo.

Culture media for embryo growth was first described in 1912 for the growth of an embryo of a rabbit. Later on in 1949, mouse embryos were grown in culture media from the 8-cells stage to blastocysts. These culture media, like Earle, Ham's F10, Tyrode's T6 and Whitten's WM1 were based on different salts and were constructed to support the development of somatic cells and cell lines in culture. These culture media, known as physiological salt solutions were used by Robert Edwards for his first successful IVF attempt. These media were formulated for use with or without serum supplementation, depending on the cell type being cultured. The Ham's Nutrient Mixtures were originally developed to support growth of several clones of Chinese hamster ovary (CHO) cells, as well as clones of HeLa and mouse L-cells.

In 1984 to 1985, special media were developed for human IVF. Menezo and his colleagues published a paper, in 1984, describing a new concept in Human Embryo culture. They suggested adding serum albumin as a source for amino acids. The serum protein ensures that oocytes and embryos do not adhere to the glass surface of the pipette used to manipulate them. The medium entitled B2, is still in use today. In 1985, Quinn et al. published in the journal Fertility and Sterility a formula entitled Human Tubal Fluid (HTF), which mimics the *in vivo* environment to which the embryo is exposed. The formulation of HTF was based on the known chemical composition of the fluids in human fallopian tubes as known at that time. This medium is based on a simple balanced salt solution without amino acids; however, the concentration of potassium was adjusted to that measured in the human female reproductive tract. This medium was found to be better compared with earlier media developed.

The supplementation of the HTF medium with either whole serum or with serum albumin became a gold standard for the production of culture medium for human embryos transferred on day 2 or day 3 of culture.

Over the years, further basic research on the metabolism of preimplantation embryos revealed that there are specific needs depending on the developmental stage of the embryo. Energy source requirements evolve from a pyruvate-lactate preference while the embryos, up to the 8-cell stage, are under maternal genetic control, to a glucose based metabolism after activation of the embryonic genome that supports their development from 8-cells to blastocysts.

The above observation lead to the development of the first commercial media. The culture media developed was based on HTF: both media were free of inorganic phosphate, glucose and amino acids. Pool and his colleagues formulated HTF which was free of glucose and phosphate.

Later experiments performed by Gardner and his colleagues supported these findings, further demonstrating the changing metabolic needs of the embryo between its cleavage stages up to 8-cells and later stages up to blastocysts. Cleaving embryos use pyrovate and lactate as energy sources and non-essential amino acids (NEAA) for protein metabolism. From the 8-cell stage the major energy source is glucose and for protein metabolism the embryos use essential amino acids (EAA). Gardner et al. also showed significant differences in the concentrations of various metabolites between the fallopian tube and the uterus.

These findings lead Gardner and his colleagues to formulate the composition of two culture media G1 and G2 that are to be used in sequence. G1 supports the *in-vitro* development of the fertilized oocyte, the zygote, to the 8-cell stage, and G2 from 8-cells to blastocyst. Several modifications to these media were formulated also by other groups. Sequential media are now being used successfully in IVF treatment all over the world.

Composition

Culture media containing a phosphate buffer or Hepes organic buffer are used for procedures that involve handling of gametes outside of the incubator, flushing of follicles and micromanipulation.

pH and Osmolality

Most culture media utilize a bicarbonate/CO_2 buffer system to keep pH in the range of 7.2 to 7.4. The osmolarity of the culture medium must be in the range of 275 to 290 mosmol/kg.

Temperature

The human oocyte is temperature-sensitive and a humidified incubator with a temperature setting of 37.0 to 37.5°C must be used for oocyte fertilization and embryo culture.

Culture Conditions

Embryos should be cultured under paraffin oil, which prevents evaporation of the medium preserving a constant osmolarity. The oil also minimizes fluctuations of pH and temperature when embryos are taken out of the incubator for microscopic assessment. Paraffin oil can be toxic to gametes and embryos; therefore, batches of oil must be screened and tested on mouse embryos before use in culture of human embryos.

Water

The medium is composed of 99% water. Purity of the water is crucial, and is achieved by ultrafiltration.

Protein Source

Albumin or synthetic serum are added in concentrations of 5 to 20% (w/v or v/v, respectively). Today, the commercial media includes synthetic serum in which the composition is well known.

Sources for Protein Supplements (serves today for research only)

- Human serum
- Human cord serum (HCS) (difficult to obtain)
- Human serum albumin (HSA)
- Fetal calf serum (FCS)
- Bovine serum albumin (BSA).

Commercial IVF Media

- Synthetic serum
- Recombinant albumin.

Salt Solution in MTF

NaCl, KCl, KH_2PO_4, $CaCl_2 . 2H_2O$, $MgSO_4 . 7H_2O$, $NaHCO_3$

Carbohydrates

Carbohydrates are present in the female reproductive tract. Their concentrations vary throughout the length of the oviduct and in the uterus, and are also dependent on the time of the cycle.

Together with the amino acids they are the main energy source for the embryo. Culture media that support the development of zygotes up to 8-cells contain pyruvate and lactate. Some commercial media are glucose free, while others add a very low concentration of glucose to supply the needs of the sperm during conventional insemination.

Media that support the development of 8-cell embryos up to the blastocyst stage contain pyruvate and lactate in low concentrations and a higher concentration of glucose.

Amino Acids

Supplement of the culture medium with amino acids is necessary for embryo development. Media that support the development of zygotes up to 8-cells are supplemented with non essential amino acids. Proline, serine, alanine, aspargine, aspartate, glycine, glutamate.

Media that support the development of 8-cell embryos up to the blastocyst stage are supplemented with essential amino acids: Cystine, histadine, isolucine, leucine, lysine, methionine, valine, argentine, glutamine, phenylalanine, therionine, tryptophane.

Vitamins

Their role in the culture medium is unclear.

Antibiotics

The majority of ART laboratories use culture media containing antibiotics to minimize the risks of microbial growth. The most commonly used antibiotics being Penicillin (β-lactam Gram-positive bacteria disturbs cell wall integrity) and Streptomycin (Aminoglycoside Gram-negative bacteria disturbs protein synthesis). The antibacterial effect of penicillin is attributed to its ability to inhibit the synthesis of peptidoglycan, unique glycoproteins of the bacterial cell wall. Streptomycin and gentamycin belong to the aminoglycoside group of antibiotics which exert their antibacterial effect by inhibiting bacterial protein synthesis. The use of gentamicin is still controversial and it is not being used by every laboratory.

Chelators

EDTA is used as a chelator in medium that supports the embryo from the zygote stage to 8-cells and prevents abnormal glycolysis.

HTF Hepes

Designed for oocyte retrieval and follical flushing. It is modified HTF formulated with EDTA and alanyl glutamine buffered with bicarbonate and hepes. It contains needed antibiotics.

Enhance HTF

Designed for *in vitro* procedure involving the culture of early cleavage stage embryo. Modified HTF formulated with EDTA, low phosphate, alanyl glutamine.

Enhance Day 1

Designed for culture of embryo from day 1 through the morula stage, day 3 or 4. It is glucose and phosphate free with the addition of EDTA and alanyl glutathione.

Enhance Day 3

Designed for culture of embryo for day 3 transfers or for Blastocyst culture. It is low glucose and phosphate free media formulated with EDTA, taurine, glutathime and alanyl glutamine.

Enhance Day 5

Designed for culture of embryo to blastocyst and day 5 embryo transfers. It is phosphate free and having elevated levels of glucose supplemented with vitamins, essential and non essential amino acids formulated with glutathione and alanyl glutamine.

Human Serum Albumin (HSA)

It is the protein of choice for use as a tissue culture supplement in those applications requiring protein supplementation. It contains 100 mg/mL total protein (wt/volume) in normal saline.

Mineral Oil

It is the recommended oil for overlaying during fertilization of embryo culture and micro-manipulation.

Polyvinyl Pyrrolidone (PVP)

It is the recommended media to decrease sperm motility for ICSI procedure prevent sperm sticking to the glass pipette.

Hyaluronidase

It is the recommended medium for removal of cumulas cells from the oocyte after egg retrieval and prior to ICSI.

2

Shubhangi Gangal

Computer-assisted Semen Analysis (CASA)

INTRODUCTION

The use of computer-assisted semen analysis (CASA) has advanced the ability to study and understand sperm function as it relates to human infertility. The major advances have been in the ability to more accurately determine sperm concentration (counts) and motility (movement). Generally, sperms are "looked" at by a computerized digitizing tablet through a microscope. The computer has been "taught" by the laboratory personnel what sperm look like, and how they move. When the computer then "sees" a sperm under the microscope, it is able to draw a digitized picture of each individual sperm, including the speed and path this sperm takes while moving under the microscope. A great deal has been learned about the normal and abnormal "micro"characteristics of sperm employing this method. The method is, however, not foolproof. The computer is only as intelligent as its programmer. Small changes in the computer program can alter the sperm calculations significantly. The computers must constantly be monitored and updated. In our laboratories, all grossly abnormal CASA assays are always verified by both a repeat analysis as well as with a "hands on" human second look opinion. We feel that any abnormal sperm count must be verified by a manual counting and assessment method.

The commercial introduction of various computer-assisted semen analysis (CASA) systems has greatly facilitated the analysis of semen in many andrology laboratories. Use of automated CASA systems eliminates subjective human errors and provides potential for accurate quantitative evaluation of semen (Figs 2.1 to 2.3).

Various CASA systems like Cell Soft (Cryo Resources Ltd, NY), Hamilton Thorne (Hamilton Thorne Research Inc, Danvers, MA), Cell Trak (Motion analysis Corp, Santa Rosa, CA) are used widely all over.

Sperm motion kinetics measured by CASA includes the following:

1. Sperm concentration
2. Percent motility
3. *Curvilinear velocity (VCL; micrometers per second):* The time-average velocity of a sperm head along its actual curvilinear path, as perceived in two dimensions in the microscope.

4. *Straight-line velocity (VSL; micrometers per second):* The time-average velocity of a sperm head along the straight line between its first detected position and its last.
5. *Average path velocity (VAP; micrometers per second):* The time-average velocity of a sperm head along its average path. This path is computed by smoothing the actual path according to algorithms in the CASA instrument: these algorithms vary between instruments.
6. *Linearity (LIN; percent):* The LIN of a curvilinear path, VSL/VCL.
7. *Amplitude of lateral head displacement (ALH; micrometers):* The magnitude of lateral displacement of a sperm head about its average path. This can be expressed as a maximum or an average of such displacement.

In addition to the computerized results, manual results are also calculated for sperm concentration and motility.

Standardization, strict quality control, and quality assurance are critical and should be strictly enforced in the program. An intra-assay variation of less than 10% was seen in CASA sperm counts and motility.

Computer-assisted semen analysis (CASA) systems couple video technology and sophisticated microcomputers for automatic image digitalization and processing. This technology was developed for more objective measurements of seminal parameters over the subjective measures of standard semen analysis.

CASA permits the measurement of additional motility parameters such as curvilinear velocity, straight-line velocity, linearity, and flagellar beat frequency. Under certain circumstances, CASA has been found to be less accurate than the standard semen analysis and the biological and clinical relevance of some of these new parameters has yet to be validated.

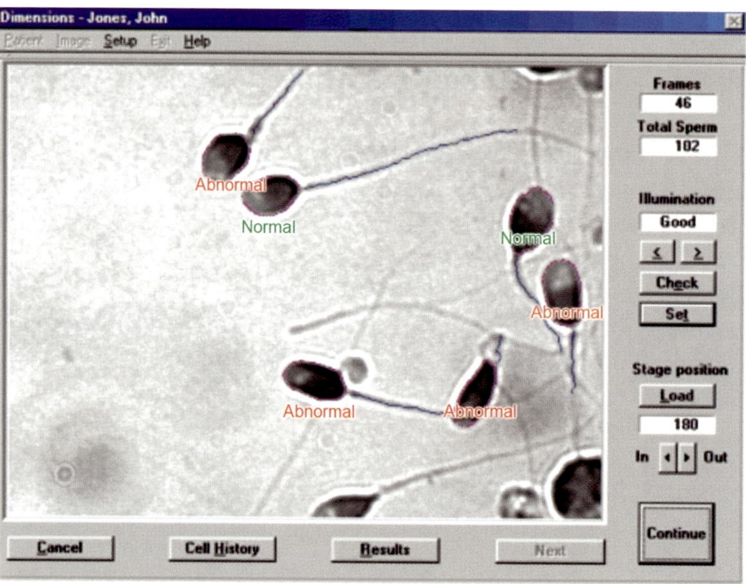

FIGURE 2.1: Sperm dimension

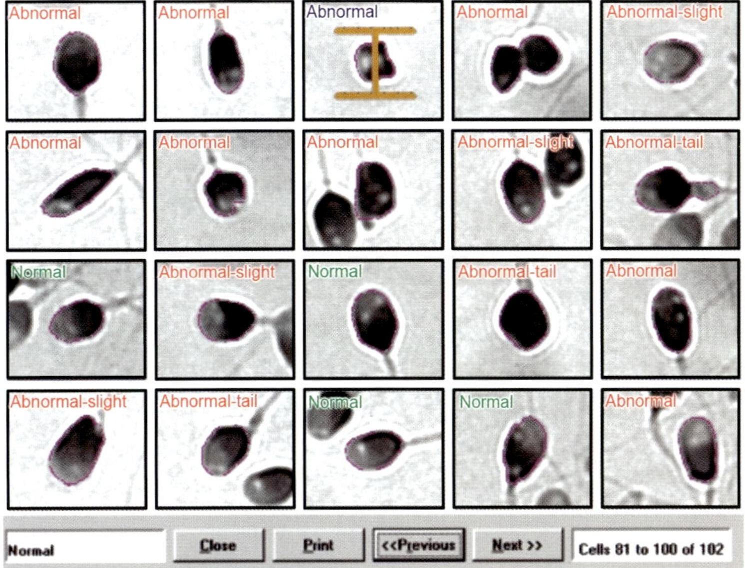

FIGURE 2.2: Head abnormalities

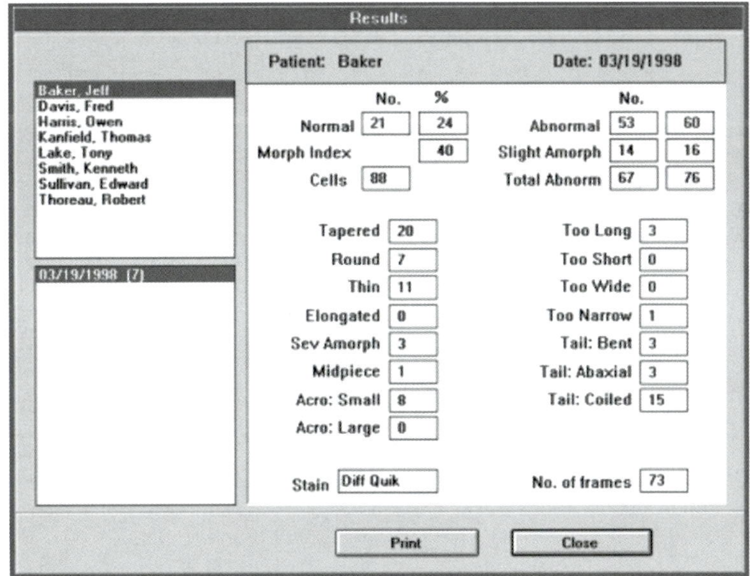

FIGURE 2.3: CASA report

Also since the equipment is very expensive and needs trained personnel to read and understand the analysis, the computer-assisted methods are still not very popular in day-to-day practice.

BIBLIOGRAPHY

1. Agarwal A, Ozturk E, Loughlin KR. Comparison of semen analysis between the two Hamilton-Thorn semen analysers. Andrologia. 1992;24:327-9.
2. Larsen L, Scheike T, Jensen TK, Bonde JP, Ernst E, Hjollund NH, et al. Computer-assisted semen analysis parameters as predictors for fertility of men from the general population. Hum Rep. 2000;15(7):1562-7.

3

Kuldeep Jain

Semen Analysis

INTRODUCTION

Semen analysis is an important "gateway test" for evaluating male infertility. It is often the 1st test ordered when a couple presents for infertility workup, as it is a noninvasive and a relatively inexpensive test.

Semen analysis is performed in two settings:

1. General pathology clinical laboratories
2. Andrology/fertility laboratories.

No matter where it is performed, it is usually unreliable. Inspite of the importance of semen analysis in diagnosis and management of male infertility, it remains "the most neglected laboratory test" in most laboratories.

Some of the possible reasons and factors responsible for unreliable and questionable reports are:

1. Training for semen analysis is minimal or inadequate in most of the time and is often not included in the clinical training at all.
2. Unlike most of the clinical pathology investigations, it relies upon values and professional judgment of the analyst, who may not be sensitive towards the implications of correct or incorrect report.
3. Most of laboratories use the procedure which is outmoded or passed on through years without any effort to modernize or validate it.
4. Semen analysis is practically the last manual microscopic test in the laboratory because of lack of an affordable, operation-friendly technology.
5. Semen analysis involves multiple parameters to be simultaneously evaluated and therefore, considerable laboratory time is consumed when is properly performed.
6. Lack of quality control benchmarks and ambiguity of methodology especially for motility and morphology.

The present chapter is an attempt to provide a step by step systemic and easy approach for a perfect semen analysis.

Semen analysis is divided into five categories:

1. Background data
2. Physical data

3. Quantitative and qualitative analysis
4. Biochemical analysis
5. Screening test.

These components are interrelated and cannot be interpreted in isolation. Facts such as days of abstinence, previous H/o drug intake, previous illness, etc. have got a direct bearing on semen analysis results.

Terminology

Spermia	Ejaculate
Aspermia	No ejaculate
Hematospermia	Blood in ejaculate
Leukocytospermia	Leukocytes in ejaculate
Zoospermia	Spermatozoa in ejaculate
Azoospermia	No sperm in semen
Normozoospermia	Normal semen parameters
Olgizoospermia	Low sperm count
Asthenozoospermia	Poor motility
Teratozoospermia	Poor morphology
Necrozoospermia	All spermatozoa dead
Globozoospermia	Round-headed sperms

Background Data

It consists of certain basic facts which should be recorded and interpreted along with semen analysis report. Method of sample collection, time of collection, time of analysis, days of abstinence, H/o smoking, alcohol and, H/o drug intake, HIV/STD/Hepatitis are all important factors that can have an influence on the result.

Container

A wide mouthed polypropylene sterile prelabelled jar is used to collect semen.

A nonlatex, sialastic condom may be used to collect semen sample during coitus.

Abstinence

Two to five days of ejaculatory abstinence is required for normal semen analysis. Long abstinence time affects almost all seminal parameters.

Method for Production

Providing a private and comfortable environment is important for successful collection of semen sample as many patients may not be able to produce semen in clinical settings. Sample is produced by masturbation or by intercourse and collected in wide mouth container without spillage. If any spillage occurs, it should be enquired and noted.

Time of sample collection should be noted. It is preferable that semen is collected at laboratory/clinic. However, if brought from home, the time elapsed during transportation should be noted.

Once the sample is received in the lab, further evaluation should be done in the following steps:

1. Check the name of patient and other details on the request form.
2. Time of sample received in lab is recorded.
3. As handling of semen sample carries the risk of exposure to infectious pathogens, protective measures such as gloves and spill resistant gowns should be used by laboratory staff.

Physical Parameters

a. *Coagulation:* Just after ejaculation, normal semen quickly transforms into a coagulum under the influence of protein kinase (Semenogelin) secreted by seminal vesicles.
   Implication: Absence of coagulum formation denotes congenital absence of vas and seminal vesicles.
b. *Liquification:* It should be evaluated at the end of 30 minutes and if incomplete, at the end of 60 minutes. Liquification is brought about by a proteolyte enzyme fibrinolysin, a product of prostate.
   Implication: It servers as an indicator of normal prostate function. Incomplete liquification may result into decreased motility as intact seminogelin immobilize sperm.
c. *Viscosity:* Viscosity is the consistency of semen after liquification. Nonliquification (non-homogeneous appearance) and viscous sample (homogenous but sticky) are different and must be distinguished. It is best tested by modified pippete and released slowly in a dropwise fashion. It is considered normal if it form single drop. If threads are formed between drops, it is considered viscous. The length of thread denotes the severity.
   Implication: Increased viscosity is the result of prostatic infection and seminal vasculitis.
   - Adverse effect on determination of sperm count and motility.
   - Can be corrected by forcing the semen through a narrow gauge needle or releasing the semen against the bottom of the container.
   - Amylase or chymotrypsin can be used to reduce viscosity.
d. *Volume:* Measuring the volume of ejaculate is important as it relates to so many conditions. The best way to measure the ejaculate volume is while checking for viscosity. Whole sample is drawn in a graduated serological pipette, the volume is noted and then checked for viscosity.
   Normal semen volume is considered 1.5 to 6 mL.
   Implication: Sample less than 1 mL is seen in congenital absence of the vas, obstruction due to infection and retrograde ejaculation.
e. *Color and odor:* While checking for volume and viscosity, semen color and odor are noted.
   Implication: An ovious unpleasant odor is indicative of infection or prolong abstinence. Brown color semen may be noticed in assisted ejaculates.
f. *pH:* pH measurement may help to differentiate between acute prostatitis/vesiculation and obstruction, where it is more than 8. While in chronic infection, pH is always below 7.2.

In cases of obstruction it is below 7. It can be measured by a calorimetric indicator paper by putting a semen drop on paper and comparing against a color scale.

Microscopic Examination

Step 1: Semen is primarily examined microscopically for presence of bacteria, round cell, debris and agglutination. This step is accomplished by a wet preparation.

Place a 10 μL drop of well-mixed semen on a glass slide and a coverslip:

Look for: amount of debris → moderate/heavy

Bacteria → presence or absence

Round cell → reported as

No./HPF (X40) or counted as absolute count (1 million/mL) as threshold for leukocytospermia.

Agglutination: Sperm to sperm
Sperms to cells or debris

(*Note:* The same can be done at the time of sperm counting using a chamber without dilution.)

Step 2: For manual sperm count, the best choice is to use counting chambers designed specifically for sperm counting. There are two distinct advantages of counting chamber. No dilution is required and they have an appropriate depth (10–20 μm) allowing the motile and dead sperms to be viewed in same plane. Many chambers like Makler, sperm cell, cell vision, cell-view and microcell are available.

Another advantage of sperm counting chamber is that counting of sperms and motility can be assessed at the same time.

Standard chamber has got a grid of 100 squares. Sperms (both motile and nonmotile) are counted in horizontal or vertical direction. Number of sperms in 10 squares give the sperm concentration, i.e. number of sperms per mL. It is recommended that at least 200 sperms should be counted to improve precision. If concentration is less, then multiple rows/columns need to be counted and then divided by number of columns/rows counted to get sperm concentration.

Total sperm count is obtained by multiplying the sperm concentration by semen volume.

Step 3: Manual assessment of motility: Assessment of motility is often complicated and time consuming and full of mistakes if is not precisely done. Reproducibility is also questionable.

An easier and much more objective method is as follows:

- Aliquet 100 μL well mixed semen in a 1 mL microvial.
- Incubate the vial at 56 °C for about 5 minutes to immobilize all sperm.
- In the meantime load fresh semen in chamber and count only the nonmotile sperm in a given field.
- Load immortalized sperm in chamber and count all the sperm in the same field. This gives the total sperm concentration also.

- The difference between total numbers of sperm minus the number of non motile sperm gives number of motile sperm. One can calculate percentage of motile sperm, concentration and absolute number of sperm with these two values. It is easier to count nonmotile sperm and this method is reproducible.

WHO classification requires grading of motility like rapid linear progression, slow progression and nonprogression. This is again done by subjective assessment though rapid moving sperm are difficult to count by human eye and often variable. A more objective assessment can be made by counting number of square each sperm swims in a given amount of time.

a. Multibutton tally is used during counting.
b. First count slow moving sperm (sperm that do not move more than one square during counting a row of square(s)).
c. Second button is used to count non moving sperms in the same row of squares (NM).
d. Now load immobilized sperms and count the number of sperms in the same row of square (T).
e. T–S + NM give number of rapid progressive sperms (RP).
f. RP/T $\times$ 100 =% of RP
   S/P $\times$ 100 =% of slow progressive.

Step 4: Sperm viability: It is done to differentiate dead from nonmotile but live sperm. A double stain is used using eosin V as stain and nigrosin as s counter stain. Sperm which take up the eosin are dead. Both can be visualized against blue-black nigrosin counter stain.

Step 5: Sperm morphology: It is one of the most predictive measure of fertility potential and therapeutic outcome. However, sperm morphology is most confusing component to perform and difficult to interpret.

One should not comment about the morphology on wett preparation as sperm requires staining to be visualized completely.

Method

- Make a good smear—not too thin—not too thick—Fix immediately with spray.
- Stain with modified Papanicolaou stain. After staining → smear is coverslipped and examined using 100x oil objective.
- Head, mid piece and tail of each sperm is evaluated, at least 200 sperm should be examined.
- If any of the three major structure is abnormal, sperm is classified as abnormal.

Training/ quality control for semen analysis: Though semen analysis is one of the most important lab test for infertility management, It is usually performed in the most casual manner and interpreted by clinician in the same way (Table 3.1).

Formal semen analysis training is rare and without adequate education, it is very difficult to feel confident about clinical test results. Many laboratories do not have budget for training. However, self-paced training courses and video are available for the laboratories that want to improve technical skills of its staff.

Lower reference limits (5th centiles and their 95% confidence intervals) for semen characteristics	
Parameter	*Lower reference limit*
Semen volume (mL)	1.5 (1.4–1.7)
Total sperm number (10^6 per ejaculate)	39 (33–46)
Sperm concentration (10^6 per mL)	15 (12–16)
Total motility (PR + NP,%)	40 (38–42)
Progressive motility (PR,%)	32 (31–34)
Vitality (live spermatozoa,%)	58 (55–63)
Sperm morphology (normal forms,%)	4 (3.0–4.0)
Other consensus threshold values	
pH	>7.2
Peroxidase-positive leukocytes (10^6 per mL)	<1.0
MAR test (motile spermatozoa with bound particles,%)	<50
Immunobead test (motile spermatozoa with bound beads,%)	<50
Seminal zinc (micromol/ejaculate)	>2.4
Seminal fructose (micromol/ejaculate)	>13
Seminal neutral glucosidase (mU/ejaculate)	>20

Source: WHO Lab. Manual 2010

BIBLIOGRAPHY

1. WHO Lab Manual for the examination and processing human semen, 5th Edition. Cambridge University Press. 2010.

Savita Nagpal

4 Sperm Morphology

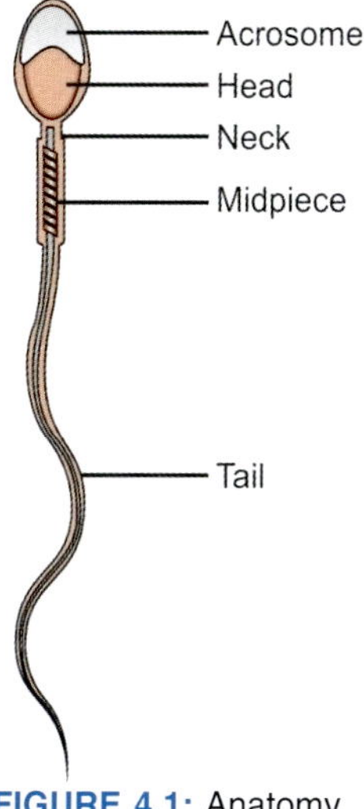

FIGURE 4.1: Anatomy of sperm

Semen analysis is a keystone in the clinical workup while estimating a man's fertility potential. It is now widely accepted that sperm morphology is the semen characteristic most correlated with fertility, and particularly with fertilizing ability *in vitro*.

The standardization of what constitutes a normal spermatozoon is essential (Fig. 4.1).

- The WHO criteria (1987, 1992).
- The strict criteria.
- Computer-assisted methods.

THE WHO CRITERIA (1987)

- Normal frequency: 50%
- Head shape: Regular oval shaped
- Head size: 3 to 5 μm long, 2 to 3 μm wide
- Length/width ratio: 1.5 to 2.0
- Acrosome: > 1/3
- Vacuoles: No details
- Cytoplasmic droplets: No details
- Midpiece: 7 to 8 μm, <1/3 width of head, slender, straight and regular, aligned with longitudinal axis of head.
- Tail: At least 45 μm, slender, uncoiled and regular.

THE WHO CRITERIA (1992)

- Normal frequency: 30%.
- Head shape: Oval; borderline forms abnormal.
- Head size: 4.0 to 5.5 μm long and 2.5 to 3.5 μm wide.
- Length/width ratio: 1.5 to 1.75.
- Acrosome: 40–70% of head area, well defined.
- Vacuoles: <20% of head area.
- Cytoplasmic droplets: < 1/3 normal head.

- Midpiece: No dimensions, no description of normal (defects only given).
- Tail: No dimensions, no description of normal (defects only).

THE STRICT CRITERIA

- Normal frequency: 14%.
- Head shape: Oval configuration with a smooth contour, borderlines forms abnormal.
- Head size: 5 to 6 µm long and 2.5 to 3.5 µm wide.
- Width/ length ratio: 1/2–3/5.
- Acrosome: 40 to 70% of the distal part of the head, well defined.
- Cytoplasmic droplets: < 1/2 normal head.
- Midpiece: 1.5 of the head length, <1 µm wide, slender and axially attached.
- Tail: 45 µm long, uniform, uncoiled, slightly thinner than the midpiece.

After 200 individual sperm are counted at a magnification of 1,000 times, the percent normal forms is calculated. According to Kruger Strict Morphology, the prognosis is based on the following scale:

≥ 15% normal	Normal range—Good prognosis
5–14% normal	Suboptimal range—Prognosis is fair to good, however, the lower the percent normal, the lower the chance of successful fertilization
0–4% normal	Poor prognosis—Will usually need IVF with intracytoplasmic sperm injection (ICSI)

Although rapid methods such as Diff-Quick might allow rapid assessments of normal forms,they cannot provide insights into all the types of morphological defects (Figs 4.2 and 4.3) that can be obtained from Papanicolaou–stained smears (Figs 4.4 to 4.9).

Computer-assisted methods:
- The method of Moruzzi (1988)
- The Perez-Sanchez system (1994).

Head shape/size defect: Large, small tapering pyriform, amorphous, vacuolated, reduced or absent acrosome, double head.

Neck and midpiece defects: Absent tail (loose head), non-inserted or bent tail, distended or abnormally thin midpiece.

Tail defects: Short, multiple, hairpin, broken, irregular width, terminal droplet, coiled.

Immature forms: Cytoplasmic droplets >1/3rd the area of a normal sperm head.

At least 100 or preferably 200 spermatozoa are evaluated.

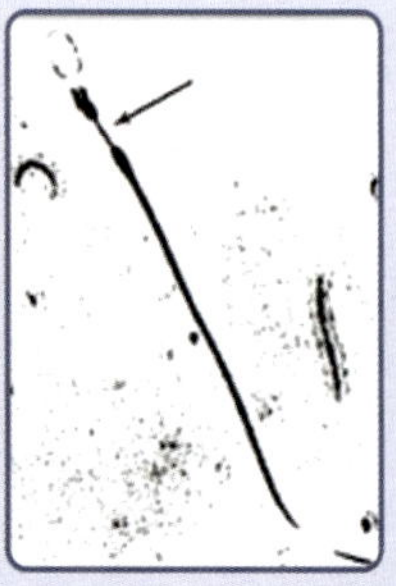

FIGURE 4.2: Morphological defects of sperm

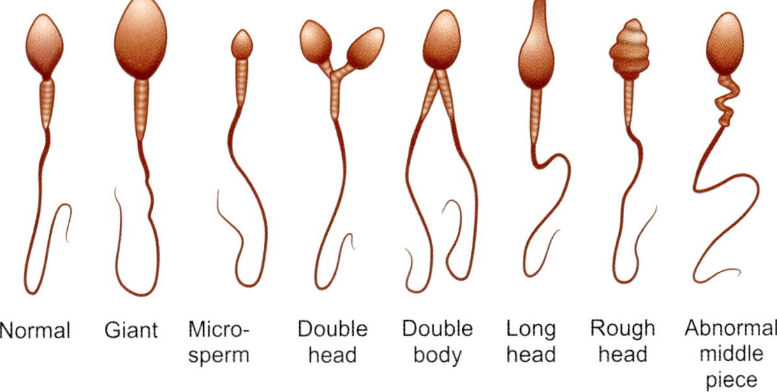

FIGURE 4.3: Sperm morphology

Initially, the traditional or so-called the liberal approach was adopted in the 1980 and 1987 WHO manual, but after the publication of strict criteria methodology in 1990, the strict criteria principles were accepted in part in the 1992 WHO manual. In the 1999 WHO manual, strict criteria became the recommended method and were confirmed as the standard method of sperm morphology evaluation in the new 2010 WHO manual (Menkveld).

Clinical Relevance of Strict Criteria

It may be argued that in itself the very low normal sperm morphology cutoff value of >4% morphological normal spermatozoa as given in the 2010 WHO manual and also in the recently published articles by Menkveld et al. and Haugen et al. may be of limited prognostic value. However, it must be kept in mind that the 2010 WHO manual cutoff value is based on the lower fifth percentile of several combined studies of so-called fertile male populations. This means that in practice most fertile men will have a higher percentage of morphologically normal spermatozoa.

However, there has been criticism on the concept and use of strict criteria from time to time, as not being scientific, not being evidence-based and unsuitable for use in the clinical laboratory. Furthermore, it was claimed that strict criteria morphology evaluations are less reproducible and less accurate than the liberal approach. In order to keep variations in sperm morphology evaluations as small as possible, it was suggested that the WHO recommendation should be changed to 'borderline normal sperm should be regarded as abnormal—or if not sure regard the sperm cells as abnormal' rather than regard it as normal (Menkveld).

Papanicolaou Stained Smear (Figs 4.5 to 4.9)

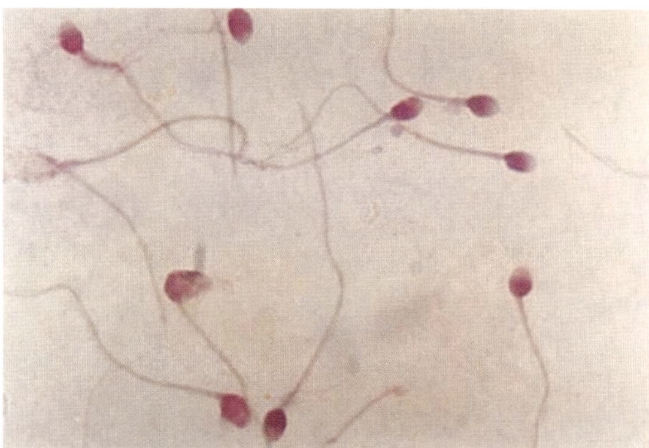

FIGURE 4.4: Normal and abnormal sperms

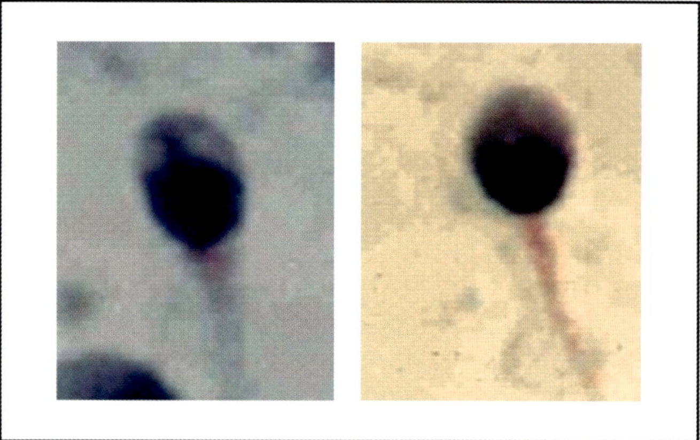

FIGURE 4.5: Normal sperm head

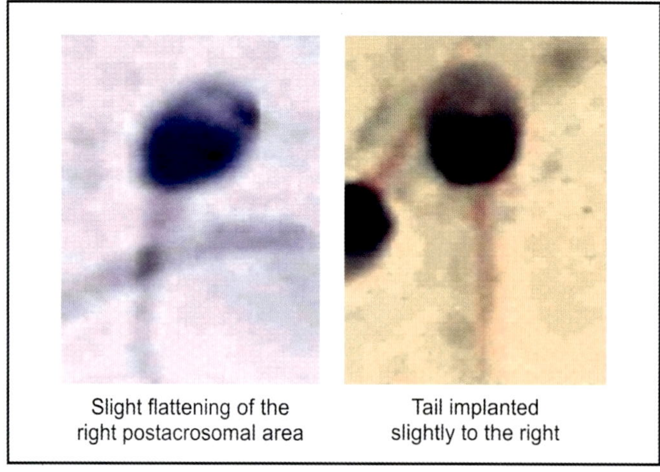

Slight flattening of the right postacrosomal area

Tail implanted slightly to the right

FIGURE 4.6: Normal variant

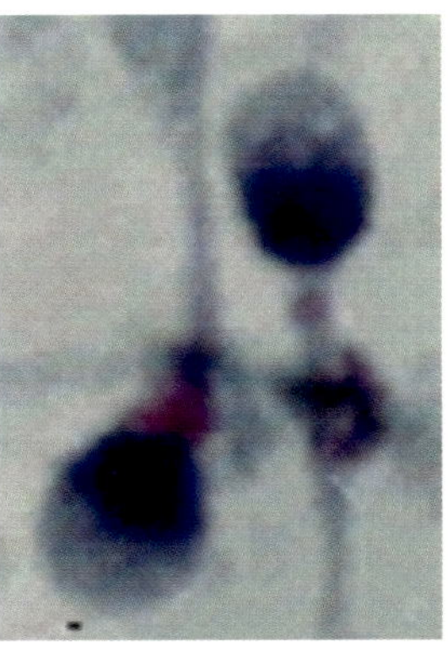

Left side spermatozoon:
Head = Abnormal due to elongated posterior of postacrosomal region.

Right side spermatozoon:
Head = Normal.
Although the right side of the postacrosomal area is slightly flattened this is not enough to classify the spermatozoon as abnormal

A

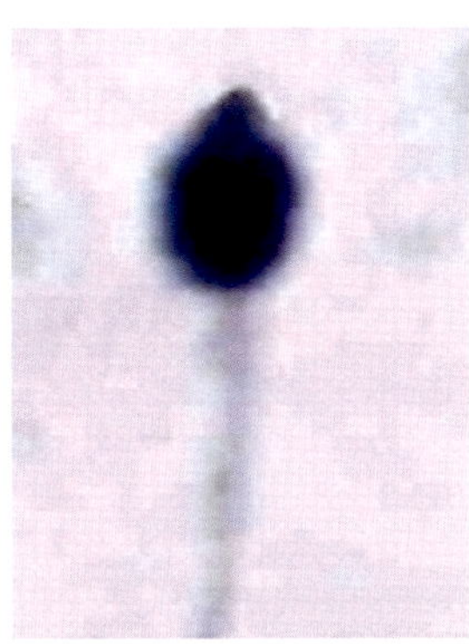

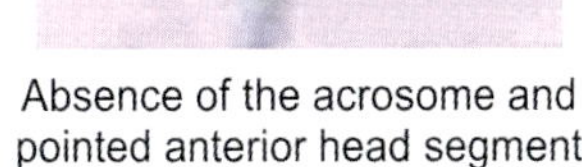

Absence of the acrosome and pointed anterior head segment

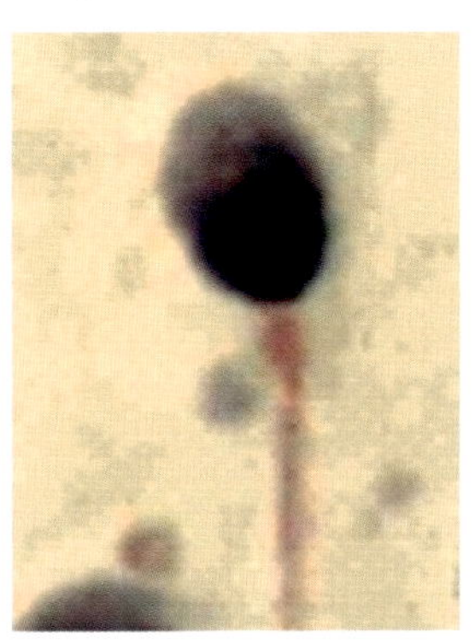

Very small acrosomal area

B

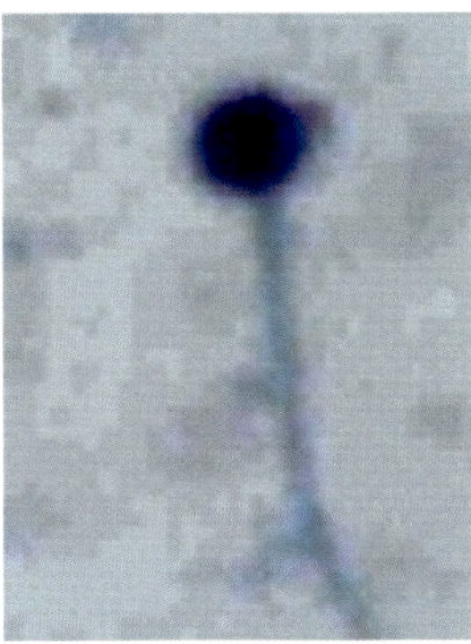

Small size and absence of acrosome with typical round-head defect or globozoospermia

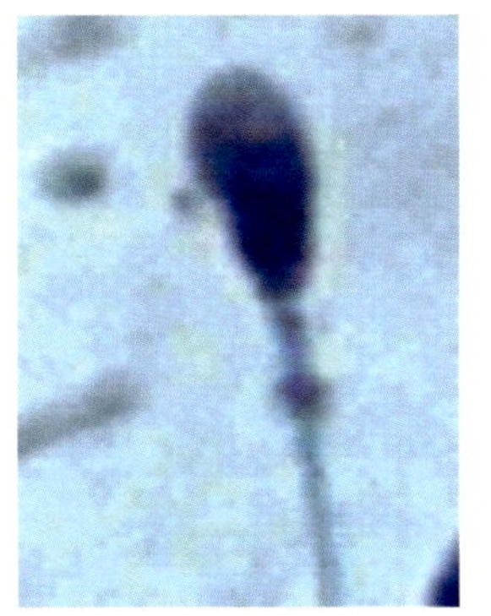

Moderate-to-severe elongation of the postacrosomal area

C

FIGURES 4.7A TO C: Abnormal sperm head

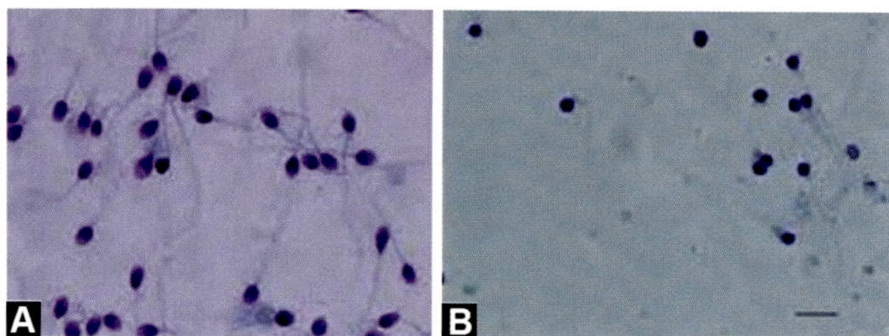

FIGURES 4.8A AND B: Globozoospermia results in the loss of the typical acrosome of normal sperm

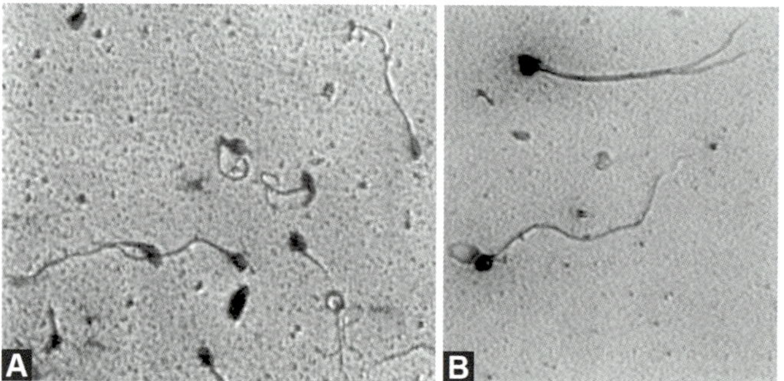

FIGURES 4.9A AND B: Fixed and stained human sperm images from our IVF lab. Some abnormal sperm morphology is shown on very high magnification

5

Sandro C Esteves

Semen Preparation: Ejaculated Sperm for ICSI

INTRODUCTION

Prolonged exposure of sperm to seminal plasma results in a marked decline in both motility and viability. Sperm incubated in synthetic culture medium free of seminal plasma contamination show no such declines. It is essential, therefore, that spermatozoa for clinical procedures such as *in vitro* fertilization (IVF)/intracytoplasmic sperm injection (ICSI) be separated from the seminal environment as soon as possible after ejaculation.

The most common methods for sperm processing are the swim-up technique and the separation through a discontinuous colloidal density gradient. Alternatively, simple washing can be employed in cases of severely oligozoospermic ejaculates. The advantage of swim-up and density gradient are that they select the sperm population exhibiting better motility, in contrast to the non-selective concentration of spermatozoa obtained through a simple wash procedure.

Sperm processing by swim-up or density gradient eliminate immotile and dead spermatozoa, along with exfoliated cells, cellular debris, and amorphous material. Sperm preparation by swim-up removes seminal plasma and concentrates the most motile spermatozoa in a very small volume of sperm culture media. However, the sperm yield is low in cases of oligozoospermic ejaculates with low motility. For this reason, swim-up is preferred for normozoospermic specimens. Conversely, density gradient centrifugation is usually preferred to process ejaculates with low sperm number, motility, or morphology, as it allows the elimination of leukocytes and other microorganisms which are trapped in the gradient interphases. Density gradients can be altered to optimize sperm recovery by decreasing the gradient volume which limit the distance that the spermatozoa migrate, or by increasing the centrifugation time in cases of hyperviscous ejaculates.

MATERIALS, EQUIPMENT AND REAGENTS

Material and Equipment

- Sterile disposable serological pipettes (1, 2, 5 and 10 mL, e.g. cat. #4051 Costar or cat. #356543 Falcon, USA)
- Disposable polystyrene conical (swim-up) and round-bottom (density gradient) centrifuge tubes (sterile) with caps.

- Disposable transfer pipets (sterile)
- Pipettor 1 to 200 µL (Gilson, France) and Sterile tips (e.g. cat. #4804, Corning, USA)
- Pipetting device (e.g. Pipette-aid, Drummond Scientific, USA)
- 6 mL sterile centrifuge polystyrene tubes with caps (e.g. cat. #352003, Falcon, USA)
- Makler Chamber
- Fine point permanent marker pen (e.g. Sharpie, Sandford, USA)
- Laminar flow cabinet
- 37°C incubator
- Centrifuge (e.g. model 225; Fisher Scientific, USA).

Reagents

- HEPES-buffered Human Tubal Fluid (e.g. Modified HTF culture medium, cat. #90126, Irvine Scientific, USA)
- Human Serum Albumin (HSA, cat. #9988, Irvine Scientific, USA)
- Colloidal density gradient (e.g. Isolate®, cat. #99264, Irvine Scientific, USA) or Pure ception® , Sage Biopharma, Bedminster, NJ. Both are colloidal suspension of silica particles stabilized with covalently bonded hydrophilic silane supplied in HEPES
    1. Lower phase (90%)
    2. Upper phase (47%).

PROCEDURES

Double-density Gradient Centrifugation

Prepare Reagents

1. Bring all components of the gradient kit (upper and lower phase) and semen samples to 37°C, for 20 minutes, in the incubator.
2. Transfer 1 mL (volume of gradient may be reduced) of the lower phase colloidal gradient into a sterile conical bottom disposable centrifuge tube.
3. Layer 1 mL upper phase on top of the lower phase using a transfer pipet. Slowly dispense the upper phase lifting the pipet up the side of the tube as the level of the upper phase rises. A distinct line separating the two layers will be observed. This two-layer gradient is stable for up to two hours.
4. Label 15 mL centrifuge tube(s) with patient's name.

Analyze and Wash Specimen

Note: Sterile techniques should be used throughout specimen processing. Sperm processing should be performed inside a Laminar flow cabinet (e.g. Class II Bio-safety cabinet)

1. Semen specimen should be allowed to liquefy completely for 15 to 30 minutes in the 37°C incubator before processing.
2. Measure volume using a sterile 5 to 10 mL pipet.

3. Remove a drop of semen using sterile technique and do a count, motility and round cell count.
   Note: Perform a pre-wash analysis. While examining the specimen, pay particular attention to extraneous round cells, debris, and bacteria that may be present. If the number of round cells are >1 million/mL, perform Endtz test immediately. A positive Endtz test should be reported to the lab director immediately.
4. Gently place up to 2 mL of liquefied semen onto the upper phase. If volume is greater than 2 mL, it may be necessary to split the specimen into two tubes before processing.
5. Centrifuge for 20 minutes at 1600 rpm.
6. The supernatant should be removed with a sterile transfer pipette to the level directly below the second layer.
7. Using a transfer pipet, add 1.5 to 2 mL of HEPES-buffered sperm wash media (HTF) and resuspend pellet. Mix gently with pipet until sperm pellet is in suspension.
   Note: Buffered-medium (HEPES or similar) is to be used with atmospheric air 37°C incubators, and the tubes' caps should be tightly closed. If the 37°C incubator atmosphere is 5% (v/v) CO_2 in air, then the medium should be buffered with sodium bicarbonate or a similar buffer, and the tubes'caps should be loose to allow gas exchange. Adherence to these principles will ensure that the culture pH is compatible with sperm survival.
8. Centrifuge for seven minutes at 1600 rpm.
9. Again, remove supernatant from the centrifuge tube using a transfer pipet down to the pellet.
10. Resuspend the final pellet in a volume of 0.5 mL using a 1 mL sterile pipet with sperm wash media (HTF). Record the final volume. Do a routine post-wash semen analysis.

Swim-up (Figs 5.1A to F)

Spermatozoa may be selected by their ability to swim out of seminal plasma and into culture medium. The semen may be diluted and centrifuged prior to swim-up, although some authors argue against this step due to the risk of peroxidative damage to the sperm membranes. Alternatively, a direct swim-up of spermatozoa from semen can be used.

A. Prepare Reagents: Bring sperm wash media to 37°C for 20 minutes in the incubator.
B. Analyze and Wash Specimen as follows:
   Note: Sterile techniques should be used throughout specimen processing.

Swim-up from a Sperm Pellet

1. Specimen should be allowed to liquefy completely for 15 to 30 minutes in the 37°C incubator before processing.
2. Measure volume using a sterile 5 to 10 mL pipet.
   Note: Perform a pre-wash analysis. While examining the specimen, pay particular attention to extraneous round cells, debris, and bacteria that may be present. If the number of round cells are > 1 million/mL, perform Endtz test immediately. A positive Endtz test should be reported to the lab director immediately.

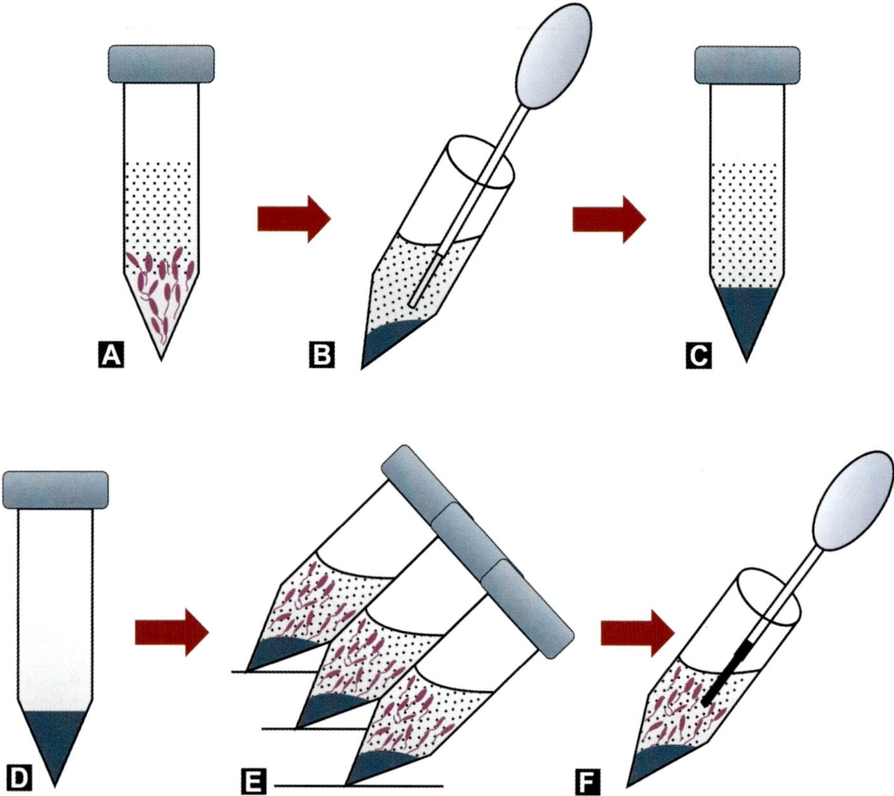

FIGURES 5.1A TO F: Swim-up from the centrifuged pellet

A. Transfer specimen from a plastic cup to a sterile 15 mL conical centrifuge tube. If specimen is >2 mL, split into two or more tubes.
   Gently mix the specimen with HEPES-buffered sperm wash media in a ratio of 1:4 by using a sterile pasteur pipet.
   Centrifuge the tubes at 1600 rpm for 10 minutes.
B. Carefully aspirate the supernatant without disturbing the pellet.
C. Resuspend the pellet in 3 mL of fresh HEPES-buffered sperm wash media (HTF). Centrifuge the tubes at 500 rpm for five minutes.
D. Discard the supernatant without disturbing the pellet and resuspend to a final volume of 600 μL of sperm medium supplemented with 5% HSA.
E. Divide the resuspended specimen in three equal aliquots of 200 μL. Underline each aliquot beneath 800 μL of protein-supplemented sperm medium in 15 mL centrifuge tubes. Incubate the tubes at 45° angle for one hour for sperm swim-up in vertical rack in a 37°C incubator.
F. After the incubation period, aspirate 600 to 700 μL supernatant from round bottom tube. Use a pasteur pipet, with the tip placed jut about the pellet surface. Pool supernatant from the two round bottom tubes into a single 15 mL conical centrifuge tube. Centrifuge the tube at 1600 rpm for seven minutes. Aspirate the supernatant from the top of the miniscus using a pasteur pipet. Resuspend the pellet in a volume of 0.5 mL protein-supplemented sperm wash media (HTF) using a 1 mL sterile pipet and keep at 37°C until ICSI. Record the final volume.

3. Transfer specimen from a plastic cup to a sterile 15 mL conical centrifuge tube. If specimen is >2 mL, split into two or more tubes.
4. Gently mix the specimen with HEPES-buffered sperm wash media in a ratio of 1:4 by using a sterile pasteur pipet.
5. Centrifuge the tubes at 1600 rpm for 10 minutes.
6. Carefully aspirate the supernatant without disturbing the pellet and resuspend the pellet in 3 mL of fresh HEPES-buffered sperm wash media (HTF).
7. Transfer the resuspended sample into two 15 mL sterile round bottom tubes using plastic pipets (1.5 mL in each).
8. Centrifuge the tubes at 500 rpm for 5 minutes.
9. Discard the supernatant without disturbing the pellet and resuspend to a final volume of 600 μL of sperm medium supplemented with 5% HSA.
10. Divide the resuspended specimen in three equal aliquots of 200 μL. Underline each aliquot beneath 800 μL of protein-supplemented sperm medium in 15 mL centrifuge tubes. *Note:* Buffered-medium (HEPES or similar) is to be used with atmospheric air 37°C incubators, and the tubes' caps should be tightly closed. If the 37°C incubator atmosphere is 5% (v/v) CO_2 in air, then the medium should be buffered with sodium bicarbonate or a similar buffer, and the tubes'caps should be loose to allow gas exchange. Adherence to these principles will ensure that the culture pH is compatible with sperm survival.
11. Incubate the tubes at 45° angle for one hour for sperm swim-up in vertical rack in a 37°C incubator.
12. After the incubation period, aspirate 600 to 700 μL supernatant from round bottom tube. Use a pasteur pipet, with the tip placed jut about the pellet surface.
13. Pool supernatant from the two round bottom tubes into a single 15 mL conical centrifuge tube. Centrifuge the tube at 1600 rpm for seven minutes.
14. Aspirate the supernatant from the top of the miniscus using a pasteur pipet.
15. Resuspend the pellet in a volume of 0.5 mL protein-supplemented sperm wash media (HTF) using a 1 mL sterile pipet and keep at 37°C until ICSI. Record the final volume.
16. Remove a small well-mixed aliquot (~0.1 mL) and make post-wash analysis.

Direct Swim-up (Figs 5.2A to E)

1. Place 1 mL of homogeneized and liquefied semen in a sterile 15 mL conical centrifuge tube, and gently layer 1.0 to 1.5 mL of protein-supplemented sperm medium over it. Alternatively, pipette the semen carefully under the supplemented culture medium.
2. Incline the tube at an angle of about 45°, to increase the surface area of the semen culture medium interface, and incubate for one hour at 37°C.
3. Gently return the tube to the upright position and remove the uppermost 1 mL of medium.
4. Dilute this with 1.5 to 2.0 mL of supplemented medium.
5. Centrifuge the tube at 1600 rpm for five minutes.
6. Aspirate the supernatant from the top of the miniscus using a pasteur pipet.
7. Resuspend the pellet in a volume of 0.5 mL protein-supplemented sperm wash media (HTF) using a 1 mL sterile pipet and keep at 37°C until ICSI. Record the final volume. Remove an aliquot for post-wash analysis.

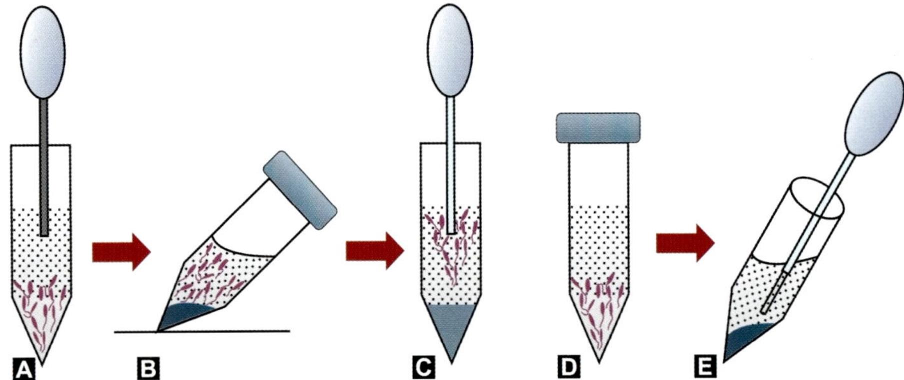

FIGURES 5.2A TO E: Direct swim-up

A. Place 1 mL of homogeneized and liquefied semen in a sterile 15 mL conical centrifuge tube, and gently layer 1.0 to 1.5 mL of protein-supplemented sperm medium over it. Alternatively, pipette the semen carefully under the supplemented culture medium.
B. Incline the tube at an angle of about 45°, to increase the surface area of the semen culture medium interface, and incubate for one hour at 37°C.
C. Gently return the tube to the upright position and remove the uppermost 1 mL of medium.
D. Dilute this with 1.5–2.0 mL of supplemented medium and centrifuge the mixture at 1600 rpm for 5 minutes.
E. Aspirate the supernatant from the top of the meniscus using a pasteur pipet. Resuspend the pellet in a volume of 0.5 mL protein-supplemented sperm wash media (HTF) using a 1 mL sterile pipet and keep at 37°C until ICSI. Record the final volume. Remove an aliquot for post-wash analysis.

BIBLIOGRAPHY

1. Esteves SC, Sharma RK, Thomas AJ Jr, Agarwal A. Effect of swim-up sperm washing and subsequent capacitation on acrosome status and functional membrane integrity of normal sperm. Int J Fertil Womens Med. 2000;45(5): 335-41.
2. Esteves SC, Sharma RK, Thomas AJ Jr, Agarwal A. Improvement in motion characteristics and acrosome status in cryopreserved human spermatozoa by swim-up processing before freezing. Hum Reprod. 2000;15(10): 2173-9.
3. Rhoden E, Soares J, Esteves S. O que o laboratório pode fazer pelo espermatozóide. II Consenso Brasileiro de Infertilidade Masculina. Int Braz J Urol. 2003;29(Suppl 5):50-55.
4. World Health Organization: WHO Laboratory Manual for the Examination and Processing of Human Semen, 5th edn. Geneva, WHO Press. 2010.p.287.

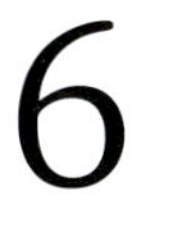

Sandro C Esteves

Semen Preparation: Sperm Extraction for ICSI

INTRODUCTION

Several sperm retrieval methods have been developed to collect epididymal and testicular sperm for ICSI in azoospermic men. As a general rule, either percutaneous epididymal sperm aspiration (PESA) or microsurgical epididymal sperm aspiration (MESA) can be successfully used to retrieve sperm from the epididymis in men with obstructive azoospermia (OA). Testicular epididymal sperm aspiration (TESA) can be used to retrieve sperm from the testes either in men with OA who fail PESA as well as in those with non-obstructive azoospermia (NOA). Testicular epididymal sperm extraction (TESE) using single or multiple open biopsies, and more recently microsurgery (micro-TESE), are indicated for men with NOA.

Processing of surgically retrieved-spermatozoa differs from the commonly used methods for processing ejaculates. Sperm processing should not only ease the selection of the best quality spermatozoa for ICSI but also optimize their fertilizing ability, whenever possible. The laboratory has a crucial role in the management of these often compromised specimens, particularly in the cases of NOA and after the freeze-thawing process. In order to achieve their goals, laboratory personnel should: (i) Receive the best quality surgically-retrieved specimen possible, with minimal or no contaminants such as red blood cells and noxious micro-organisms, (ii) Minimize the iatrogenic cellular damage during sperm processing by mastering technical skills and controlling several factors, including centrifugation force and duration, exposure to ultraviolet light and temperature variation, laboratory air quality conditions, dilution and washing steps, quality of reagents, culture media and disposable materials, and (iii) Improve the sperm fertilizing potential, if possible, by using stimulants or selecting viable sperm for ICSI when only immotile spermatozoa is available.

MATERIALS, EQUIPMENT, REAGENTS AND *IN VITRO* FERTILIZATION (IVF) LABORATORY SET-UP

Material and Equipment

- 50 × 09 mm and (e.g. #351006, Falcon, USA)
- 60 × 15 mm petri well dishes (e.g. cat. #353037, Falcon, USA; for TESA/TESE only)
- Disposable serological pipettes (e.g. 5.0 mL; cat. #4051 Costar or cat. #356543 Falcon, USA)

- Pipettor 1 to 200 μL and sterile tips (e.g. cat. #4804, Corning, USA)
- Pipetting device (e.g. Pipette-aid, Drummond Scientific, USA)
- 6 mL sterile centrifuge polystyrene tubes with caps (e.g. cat. #352003, Falcon, USA)
- 0.7 × 25 mm needles and tuberculin syringes (for TESA/TESE only)
- Fine point permanent marker pen (e.g. Sharpie, Sandford, USA)
- Injection micropipettes (e.g. cat. #MIC-50-35; Humagen, USA)
- Laminar flow cabinet
- Warming plates (e.g. Tokai-heat, Japan)
- Stereomicroscope (e.g. Leica GZ7, Switzerland)
- Centrifuge (e.g. model 225; Fisher Scientific, USA)
- Inverted microscope (e.g. Eclipse E400, Nikon, Japan) equipped with Hoffman modulation contrast and electro-hydraulic micromanipulators (Narishighe, Japan).

Reagents

- HEPES-buffered Human Tubal Fluid (Modified HTF culture medium, cat. #90126, Irvine Scientific, USA) and Human Serum Albumin (HSA, cat. #9988, Irvine Scientific, USA)
- Mineral oil (e.g. #9305, Irvine Scientific, USA)
- PVP solution (e.g. cat. #10111, Vitrolife, Sweden)
- Colloidal density gradient (e.g. Isolate®, cat. #99264, Irvine Scientific, USA).

Laboratory Set-up

Note: Use sterile handling conditions under a laminar flow cabinet or cleanroom environment during all laboratory steps.

1. Prepare a 10 mL (for PESA/MESA) or 20 mL (TESA/TESE) HEPES-buffered protein-supplemented (5% HSA) sperm culture medium, and keep it at 37°C.
2. Transfer a 5 mL aliquot of the prepared sperm culture medium to a 6 mL polystyrene tube and send it to the operating room (sperm media is used to flush the aspirating system before aspiration and to incubate epididymal aspirates or testicular specimens upon collection).
3. Place two 50 × 09 mm petri dishes on a warm surface (37°C) inside the workstation (for PESA/MESA only).
4. Prepare four 2-well dishes by transferring 0.5 mL and 1.0 mL sperm medium-aliquots to the inner and outer-dish wells, respectively (for TESA/TESE only). Place two of them onto a warm surface (37°C) inside the workstation, and send the others to the operating room (for TESE only).
5. Mount two tuberculin syringes connected with 13-gauge (to be used as tools for mincing and squeezing seminiferous tubules in TESA/TESE processing).

PESA/MESA SPERM PROCESSING (FIG. 6.1)

1. Homogenize epididymal aspirate and sperm medium to avoid sperm agglutination (epididymal spermatozoa tend to agglutinate fast). Keep aspirates-containing tubes capped at 37°C.

PESA-MESA-TESA-TESE SPERM PROCESSING

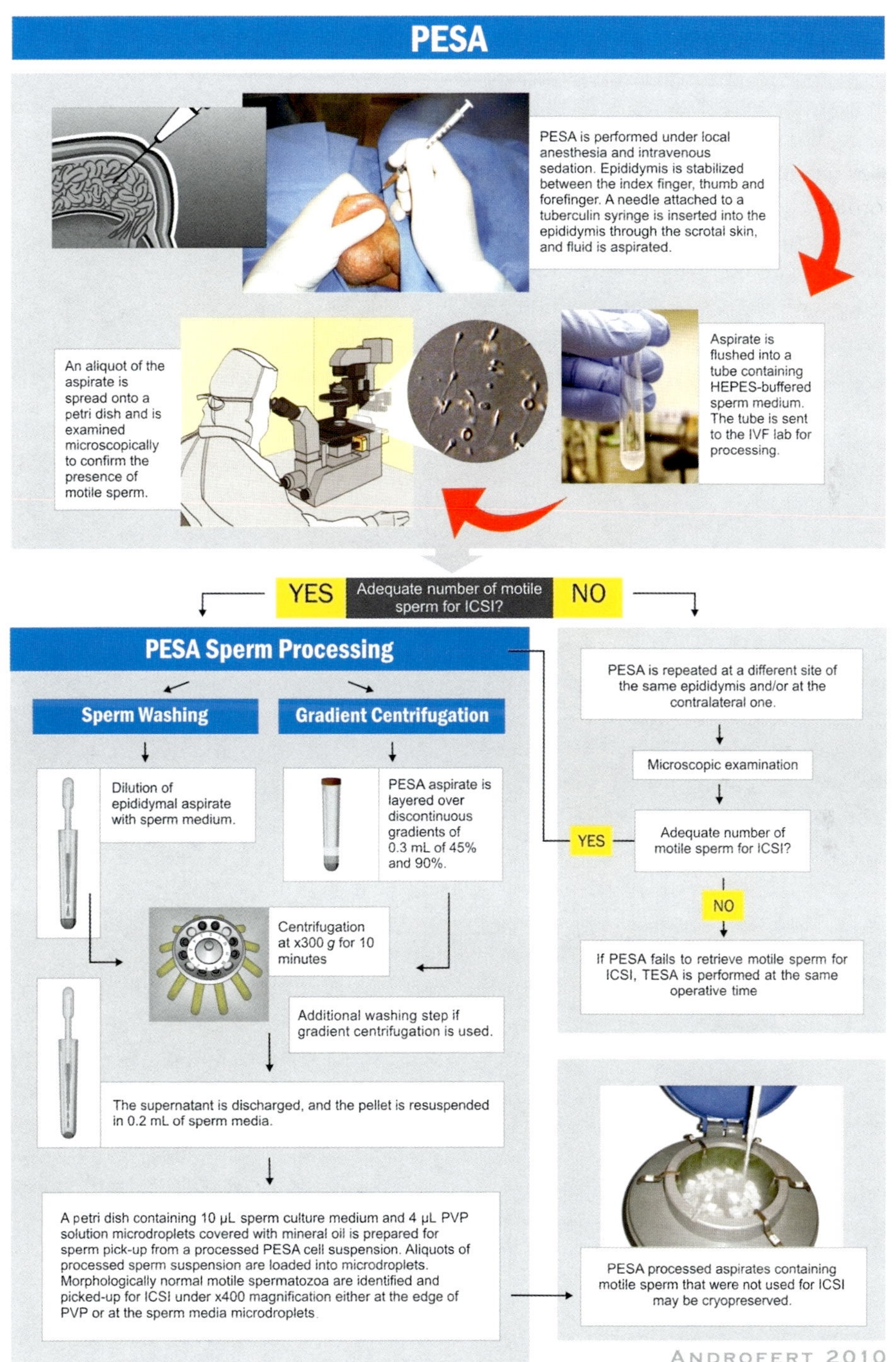

FIGURE 6.1: Percutaneous epididymal sperm aspiration (PESA)

2. Place a 10 to 20 µL mixture-aliquot onto a petri dish and spread it as thin as possible using a micropipette tip. Examine the fluid under the inverted microscope (x400 magnification) to confirm the presence of motile sperm. Inform the surgeon promptly if an adequate number of motile sperm for ICSI is available. This step should take no more than 2 to 3 minutes because the patient is kept under anesthesia until a decision of continuing or finishing the surgical retrieval is made. If more PESA specimens are taken, pool samples of similar quality together for processing. If TESA specimens are obtained, process specimens according to the "TESA processing protocol".
3. Upon finishing surgical retrieval, identify aspirate-containing tube(s) according to the epididymis side and site of aspiration, as well as to the presence of motile sperm. Make a decision upon the processing method to be used, i.e. simple washing or two-layer discontinuous mini-gradient centrifugation, based on a gross estimate of sperm density and motility. Use gradient centrifugation when the specimen contains a high density of motile sperm, particularly if contaminated with red blood cells, cellular debris and immotile sperm. Otherwise, use simple washing.
4. For density gradient centrifugation, layer an aliquot of the PESA/MESA aspirate up to 0.5 mL over 0.3 mL-gradients of 45% and 90%, respectively, and centrifuge at x300 g for 10 minutes. Resuspend the pellet in 1.5 mL fresh sperm medium and repeat centrifugation. Remove the supernatant carefully, leaving about 0.2 mL of medium above the pellet. Resuspend the pellet and keep at 37°C until use.
5. For simple washing, dilute epididymal aspirate with fresh sperm medium to a final volume of 1.5 to 2.0 mL. Centrifuge the mixture at x300 g for 10 minutes, discharge the supernatant, and then resuspend the pellet in 0.2 mL of sperm medium. When a processed PESA/MESA sample is still contaminated with an excessive number of red blood cells, dilution and centrifugation with 2 mL erythrocyte lising buffer may be required (see Appendix).
6. Prepare a petri dish containing a series of microdrops under mineral oil for sperm pick-up from a processed epididymal cell suspension.
7. Load gently a 1 µL sperm suspension aliquot at the center of the polyvinylpyrrolidone (PVP) if the sperm suspension contains motile sperm with progressive motility. After 10 to 20 minutes incubation period, morphologically normal motile spermatozoa can be identified and picked up for ICSI with the injection micropipette under x400 magnification at the edge of the PVP droplet. If progressive motility is low or absent and/or the sample is contaminated with cellular debris, load 1 to 4 µL sperm suspension aliquot at each 10 µL peripheral microdroplet of HEPES-buffered culture medium to facilitate search and selection of motile sperm. First aspirate a small volume of PVP into the injection micropipette to improve control during sperm pick-up and to avoid blowing air bubbles during ejection of selected sperm into the PVP droplet.
8. After finishing to pick-up sperm from the PESA/MESA processed sample, wash the injection micropipette free of any debris in the PVP droplet.
9. Make a final morphologic sperm assessment under x800 magnification in the group of preselected spermatozoa for ICSI. Immobilize, aspirate into the micropipette and inject selected sperm into the cytoplasm of metaphase-II oocytes.

10. Consider cryopreservation of left-over PESA/MESA processed aspirates containing motile sperm that were not used for ICSI. Freezing can be carried out using the fast liquid nitrogen vapor method.

TESA SPERM PROCESSING (FIG. 6.2)

1. Discharge TESA aspirate to the outer-dish well. Under stereomicroscopy, identify seminiferous tubules and remove blood clots using the needled-tuberculin syringes.
2. Transfer seminiferous tubules to the inner-dish well containing fresh sperm medium. Perform a mechanical dispersion of the tubules by mincing repeatedly using both needled-tuberculin syringes (use one to hold tubules in place at the bottom of the dish and the other to squeeze and open them). Repeat this step until no intact tubules are seen.
3. Examine the homogenate to confirm the presence of sperm using the inverted microscope at x400 magnification. Inform the surgeon promptly if an adequate number of sperm for ICSI is available. This step should take no more than 10 minutes because the patient is kept under anesthesia until a decision of continuing or finishing the surgical retrieval is made. If other TESA specimens are taken, carry out the initial processing steps described above. If TESE specimens are obtained, perform processing according to the "TESE sperm processing protocol" (see TESE sperm processing).
4. Aspirate and transfer the cell suspension from the inner-well dish to a sterile centrifuge tube. Dilute the aspirate with 3 mL of fresh sperm medium and wash it at x300 g for seven minutes. Discharge the supernatant and resuspend the pellet in 0.2 mL of sperm medium. When a processed TESA specimen is still contaminated with an excessive number of red blood cells, dilution and centrifugation with erythrocyte lising buffer may be required (see Appendix).
5. Prepare a petri dish as described in the "PESA/MESA protocol" for sperm pick-up from a processed testicular cell suspension.
6. Load 1 to 2 µL sperm suspension aliquot at each 10 µL peripheral microdroplet of HEPES-buffered culture medium to facilitate sperm search and pick-up. Proceed to sperm selection and ICSI, as described in the "PESA/MESA protocol", and consider cryopreservation of left-over testicular aspirates. Dishes with microdroplets containing TESA processed sperm can be incubated up to 48 hours before ICSI at room temperature in an attempt to improve testicular sperm motility.

TESE SPERM PROCESSING (FIG. 6.3)

1. Transfer TESE fragments from the operating room dishes to the outer-well of a new dish in the IVF lab. Under stereomicroscopy, remove blood clots using the needled-tuberculin syringes. Transfer fragments to the inner-well dish containing fresh medium and wash again until no blood clots are seen. Repeat these steps using new dishes if necessary, and make sure to start the mincing steps only when erythrocyte contamination is minimum (TESE fragments tend to be contaminated with excessive red blood cells).
2. Perform mechanical dispersion of the tubules, and follow the steps described in the "TESA protocol". Two laboratory technicians/embryologists should work together to speed up the

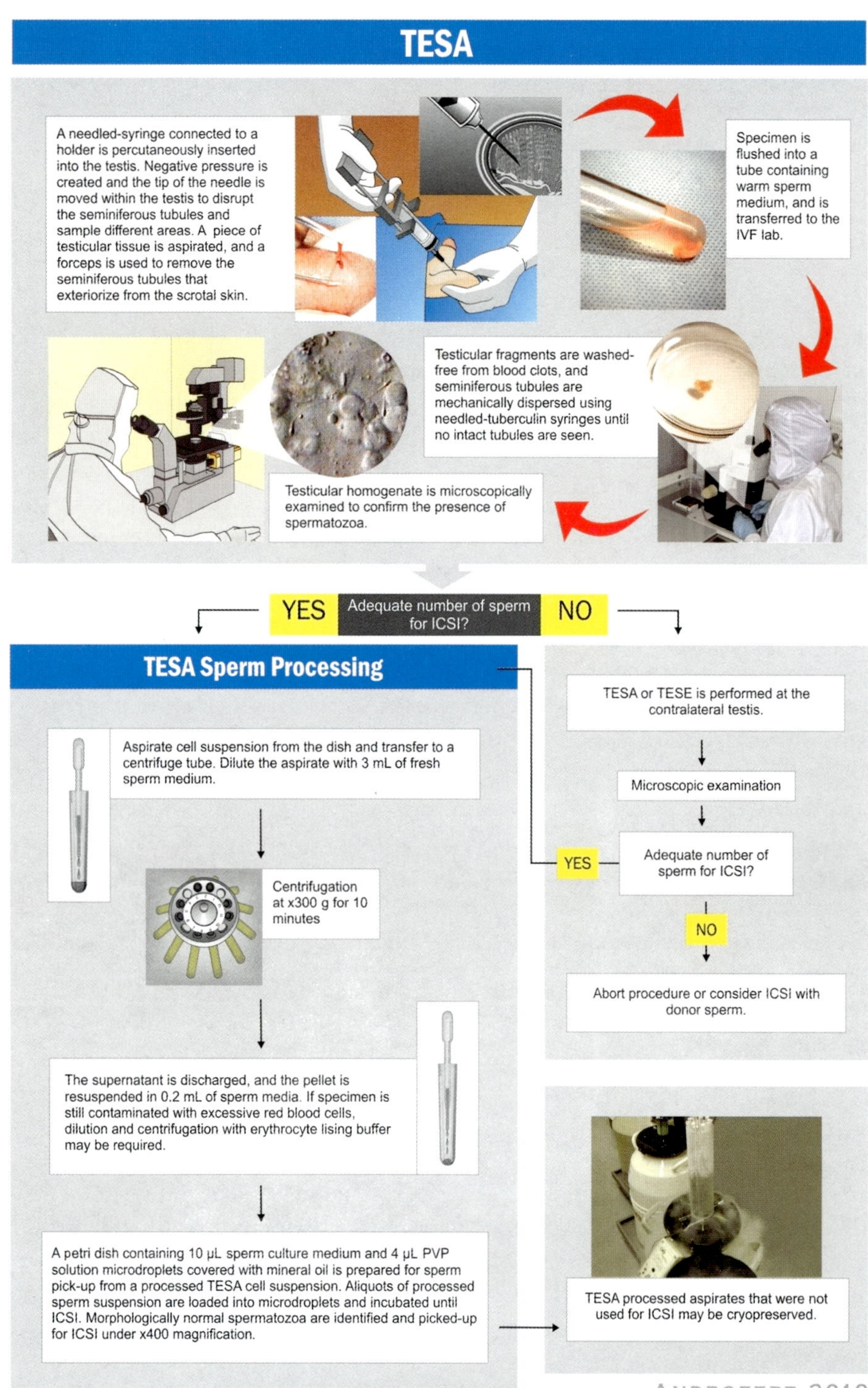

FIGURE 6.2: Testicular sperm aspiration (TESA)

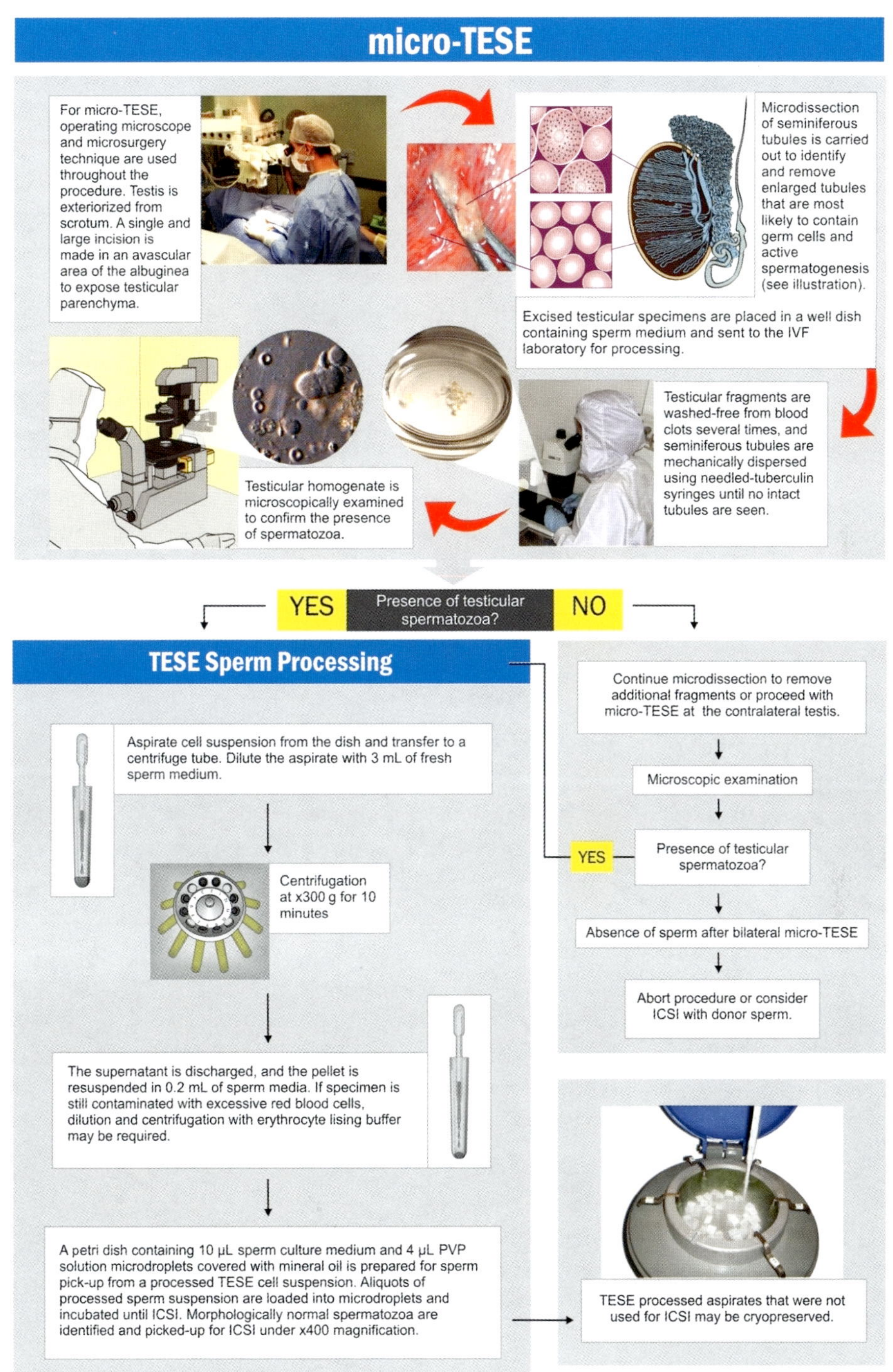

FIGURE 6.3: Testicular sperm extraction (TESE)

sperm searching process (one mincing the tubules under the stereomicroscope and the other searching for spermatozoa under the inverted microscope). Inform the surgeon promptly if any sperm is found to allow him to decide upon continuing testicular microdissection or moving to the contralateral testis. If other TESE specimens are taken, carry out the initial processing steps described above.

CRYO-THAWED EPIDIDYMAL/TESTICULAR SPERM PROCESSING

Epididymal and testicular spermatozoa may be cryopreserved using protocols routinely used for ejaculated sperm. After thawing, removal of cryoprotectant is carried out by simple washing, as described in the "TESA sperm processing protocol". If only immotile spermatozoa are seen, a method for selecting viable sperm for ICSI may be used.

METHODS FOR SELECTING VIABLE IMMOTILE SPERM FOR ICSI

It has been observed that conventional seminal parameters have little or no influence in ICSI outcomes, except when only immotile spermatozoa are available. In certain cases, only immotile spermatozoa are obtained after fresh or cryo-thawed PESA/MESA/TESA/TESE processing. Different strategies may be used to differentiate live immotile spermatozoa from dead ones, thus aiding in the selection of viable gametes for ICSI, as described below.

Hypo-osmotic Swelling Test (HOST)

1. Using the microinjection pipette, pick up morphologically normal immotile spermatozoa from the sperm medium droplet and transfer to PVP.
2. Aspirate a single spermatozoon head-first into the pipette.
3. Move the pipette to the HOS microdrop and release only the sperm tail into the HOS solution. Keep it for 5 to 10 seconds and observe if a tail tip swelling occurs (sperm tail swelling is often minimal and is a marker of viability in fresh specimens, but may not be suitable for testing cryopreserved ones).
4. If tail swelling is seen, aspirate the cell back to the pipette and release it in a drop of fresh medium to allow osmotic re-equilibration (tail swelling often disappears in 5–20 seconds). If tail swelling is not seen, discharge spermatozoon into the HOS solution.
5. Transfer the viable selected spermatozoon to the PVP drop. Repeat these steps until sufficient number of viable sperm is selected for ICSI.

Sperm Tail Flexibility Test (STFT)

1. Using the microinjection pipette, pick-up morphologically normal immotile spermatozoa from sperm microdroplet and transfer to PVP solution.
2. Align spermatozoa near the PVP droplet edge.
3. Touch sperm tail with the tip of the microinjection pipette, and force the tail to move up and down. Tail is considered flexible when it moves independently of the sperm head (sperm tail flexibility is considered a marker of sperm viability). If tail remains rigid upon

touching and sperm head and tail move together as a unit, then spermatozoon is considered non-viable for ICSI.

4. Repeat these steps until sufficient number of viable sperm is selected for ICSI.

Motility Stimulant Sperm Challenge (MSC)

Note: Example given using a 5 mM Pentoxifylline (PF) solution (see Appendix).

1. Load a 4 µL-aliquot of fresh or cryopreserved PESA/TESA/TESE sperm suspension into the motility stimulant solution microdroplet and incubate for 20 minutes.
2. Examine the specimen microscopically to search for moving sperm. In cases of a positive MSC, a slight noticeable tail twitching is often seen (in rare occasions vigorous twisting may be observed).
3. Pick-up motile sperm using the microinjection pipette and transfer to a fresh microdroplet of sperm medium. Repeat this step 3 to 4x to wash out any residual PF solution (PF was shown to be embryotoxic in animal studies, but is apparently safe if used only on sperm).
4. Keep selected spermatozoa in culture or place them into a PVP droplet for sperm selection and immobilization for ICSI.
5. Repeat these steps until sufficient number of viable sperm is selected for ICSI.

Preparation of Microdroplets

A 50 × 09 mm petri dish containing several microdroplets of culture medium under mineral oil is prepared for sperm pick-up from a processed epididymal or testicular cell suspension. Microdroplets are prepared as follows: four 10 µL sperm medium at dish periphery to load specimens (numbered 1 to 4), one 4 µL polyvinylpyrrolidone (PVP) at dish center in a triangle shape to pick-up selected sperm for ICSI (number 5), and two to three 10 µL sperm medium at dish center below the PVP triangle for washing (numbered 6 to 8). Alternatively, one of the sperm medium-containing microdroplets (e.g. number 8) or the peripheric ones (1–4) may be replaced with the hypo-osmotic or motility stimulant solutions, respectively (left). The hypo-osmotic swelling test is illustrated (right). The sperm tail is partially withdrawn from the injection micropipette into the HOS droplet. A swelling at the level of the tail tip may be seen under the inverted microscope with contrast at x400 magnification (Fig. 6.4).

APPENDIX

Erythrocyte Lising Buffer Solution (ELBS): 155 mM NH_4Cl + 10 mM $KHCO_3$ + 2 mM EDTA dissolved in sterile water. Adjust the pH to 7.2, if necessary. Upon finishing the first dilution and centrifugation step, resuspend the pellet with 2.0 mL of ELBS and keep the mixture at room temperature for 10 minutes. Then, centrifuge the sample at x300 *g* for five minutes, discharge the supernatant and resuspend the pellet in 0.2 mL of fresh HEPES-buffered protein-supplemented sperm medium.

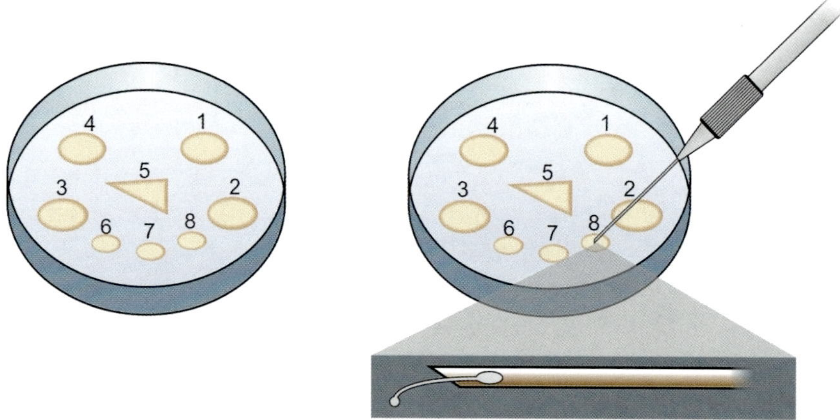

FIGURE 6.4: Preparation of microdroplets and selection of viable spermatozoa using the HOST

Hypo-osmotic Solution (HOS): Prepare a 150 mOsm/kg HOS solution by dissolving 7.35 mg sodium citrate and 13.51 mg fructose in 1 mL sterile reagent water 21. Alternatively, a 139 mOsm/kg HOS solution can be prepared by mixing 1 mL sperm medium to 1 mL sterile reagent water.

Pentoxifylline Solution (PFS): Prepare a 5 mM solution of PF by dissolving 1.391 mg pentofifylline (Sigma cat. no. P-1784) in 1 mL of HEPES-buffered culture medium.

GLOSSARY

Intracytoplasmic Sperm Injection (ICSI): A procedure in which a single spermatozoon is injected into the oocyte cytoplasm.

Azoospermia: Absence of spermatozoa in the microscopic examination of the seminal fluid after centrifugation on at least two separate occasions.

Percutaneous Epididymal Sperm Aspiration (PESA): A procedure in which a needle is inserted into the epididymis to retrieve spermatozoa for use in an ICSI procedure.

Microsurgical Epididymal Sperm Aspiration (MESA): A microsurgical procedure used to aspirate spermatozoa directly from the epididymal tubules for use in an ICSI procedure.

Testicular Sperm Aspiration (TESA): A procedure in which a needle is inserted into the testis in order to retrieve spermatozoa for use in an ICSI procedure.

Testicular Sperm Extraction (TESE): Operative removal of testicular tissue in an attempt to collect sperm for use in an ICSI procedure.

Microdissection Testicular Sperm Extraction (Micro-TESE): A microsurgical procedure used to dissect the seminiferous tubules within the testis in an attempt to identify areas of sperm production and extract spermatozoa for use in an ICSI procedure.

Sperm Processing: Laboratory techniques used to remove contaminants (cellular debris, micro-organisms, red blood cells, etc.) and to select the best quality spermatozoa to be used in conjunction to assisted reproduction technology.

Cryopreservation: The freezing process for storage of gametes or gonadal tissue at ultra-low temperature.

BIBLIOGRAPHY

1. Dafopoulos K, Griesinger G, Schultze-Mosgau A, et al. Factors affecting outcome after ICSI with spermatozoa retrieved from cryopreserved testicular tissue in non-obstructive azoospermia. Reprod Biomed Online. 2005;10:455-60.
2. Esteves SC, Sharma RK, Thomas AJ Jr, et al. Cryopreservation of human spermatozoa with pentoxifylline improves the post-thaw agonist-induced acrosome reaction rate. Hum Reprod. 1998; 13:3384-9.
3. Esteves SC, Sharma RK, Thomas AJ, et al. Improvement in motion characteristics and acrosome status in cryopreserved spermatozoa by swim-up processing before freezing. Hum Reprod. 2000;15:2173-9.
4. Esteves SC, Sharma RK, Thomas AJ Jr, et al. Suitability of the hypo-osmotic swelling test for assessing the viability of cryopreserved sperm. Fertil Steril. 1996;66:798-804.
5. Esteves SC, Spaine DM, Cedenho AP. Effects of pentoxifylline treatment before freezing on motility, viability and acrosome status of poor quality human spermatozoa cryopreserved by the liquid nitrogen vapor method. Braz J Med Biol Res. 2007;40:985-92.
6. Esteves SC, Verza Jr S. PESA/TESA/TESE sperm processing. In: Agarwal A, Varghese A, Nagy ZP (Eds). Practical methods of *in vitro* fertilization: advanced methods and novel devices. Springer, NY, in press.
7. Kovacic B, Vlaisavljevic V, Reljic M. Clinical use of pentoxifylline for activation of immotile testicular sperm before ICSI in patients with azoospermia. J Androl. 2006;27:45-52.
8. Liu J, Tsai YL, Katz E, et al. High fertilization rate obtained after intracytoplasmic sperm injection with 100% no motile spermatozoa selected by using a simple modified hypo-osmotic swelling test. Fertil Steril. 1997;68:373-5.
9. Nagy ZP, Liu J, Joris H, et al. The result of intracytoplasmic sperm injection is not related to any of the three basic sperm parameters. Hum Reprod. 1995;10:1123-9.
10. Sallam HN, Farrag A, Agameya AF, et al. The use of the modified hypo-osmotic swelling test for the selection of immotile testicular spermatozoa in patients treated with ICSI: a randomized controlled study. Hum Reprod. 2005;20:3435-40.
11. Soares JB, Glina S, Antunes N Jr, et al. Sperm tail flexibility test: a simple test for selecting viable spermatozoa for intracytoplasmic sperm injection from semen samples without motile spermatozoa. Rev Hosp Clin Fac Med Sao Paulo. 2003;58:250-3.
12. Oliveira NM, Sanchez RV, Fiesta SR, et al. Pregnancy with frozen-thawed and fresh testicular biopsy after motile and immotile sperm microinjection, using the mechanical touch technique to assess viability. Hum Reprod. 2004;19:262-5.
13. Terriou P, Hans E, Giorgetti C, et al. Pentoxifylline initiates motility in spontaneously immotile epididymal and testicular spermatozoa and allows normal fertilization, pregnancy, and birth after intracytoplasmic sperm injection. J Assist Reprod Genet. 2000;17:194-9.
14. Verheyan G, De Croo I, Tournaye H, et al. Comparison of four mechanical methods to retrieve spermatozoa from testicular tissue. Hum Reprod. 1995;10:2956-9.
15. Verza Jr S, Feijo CM, Esteves SC. Resistance of Human Spermatozoa to Cryoinjury in Repeated Cycles of Thaw-Refreezing. Int Braz J Urol. 2009;35:581-91.
16. Yovich JL. Pentoxifylline: actions and applications in assisted reproduction Hum Reprod. 1993;8:1786-91.

Ved Prakash

7 Semen Preparation: Infected Sample (HIV)

INTRODUCTION

In recent years, interest in the reproductive desire of patients who are carriers of chronic viral diseases, primarily HIV but also HCV, has increased. This interest has opened a new fields in assisted reproduction: New indications (in the case of fertile sero-different couples with the objective of semen decontamination), new adaptations of the technology for sperm preparation, new viral detection methods adapted to semen, adapted laboratories specially designed for viral hazards and new risks management.

Sexually transmitted diseases, and, among them, viruses, have always preoccupied teams practising medically assisted reproduction techniques, but mainly as a threat that should be avoided as much as possible. Contamination of patients has been described for hepatitis B virus (HBV), hepatitis C (HCV) and human immunodeficiency virus (HIV) in the last 20 years.[1] Infection with human immunodeficiency virus (HIV) affects approximately 33 million people worldwide, over 80% of whom are of reproductive age. Until the 1990s, HIV infection was an absolute contraindication to pregnancy, and couples where the man was HIV positive were not considered eligible for assisted reproduction technology (ART).[2]

Major advances in pharmaceutical research have greatly improved the prognosis of patients with HIV infection. Correct clinical and therapeutic management of these patients enables the disease to be maintained in a chronic state, in most cases avoiding fatal progression.[3]

The general condition and life expectancy of many patients with HIV infection is very good, and a percentage of young couples can be expected to make plans for the future and to want to have children. Sexual transmission of HIV is variable and depends on many different factors, such as the number of sexual partners, rather than on the frequency of sexual intercourse. Male-to-female transmission of HIV is estimated to be 1 per 1000 acts of unprotected intercourse and even less in HCV-infected patients. The presence of HCV in semen is controversial: some authors have reported a total absence of HCV RNA in semen,[4] while others suggest that HCV may be found in the semen with low or high prevalence. Levy et al.[5] identified HCV RNA in semen of HCV-infected patients.

Assisted reproductive technology with semen washing can offer a significant reduction in risk of sexual and vertical transmission of human immunodeficiency virus (HIV) and hepatitis C virus (HCV) in serodiscordant couples with infected male partner. Semprini et al. were the first to use washed sperm of HIV-1-infected men for intrauterine insemination (IUI). His team reported 2000 inseminations and 100 IVF or ICSI cycles (HIV-positive male and HIV-negative female) using their swim-up method, with a total of 350 babies born without viral contamination in 2001. However, their method may be suboptimal because it has not been proven to remove HIV RNA completely, and they did not measure proviral DNA in infected cells in the semen.[6]

RISK OF TRANSMISSION

Advances in semen preparation were followed by the use of intrauterine insemination (IUI) in HIV serodiscordant couples, which resulted in a low risk of transmission. Other studies reported the use of alternative techniques such as *in vitro* fertilization (IVF) and intracytoplasmic sperm injection (ICSI) to reduce the risk of HIV exposure to the woman and to the gamete. Although some studies have suggested that ART can be used, there is still controversy regarding the safety and effectiveness of these methods; to date, there has been no systematic review to support the use of ART in HIV serodiscordant couples.[7] In an HIV serodiscordant couple where the man is HIV positive, the risk of the woman becoming infected through unprotected sex is 0.1% to 0.2%. The couple should be informed of this risk and of the treatment options available to provide a reasonable chance of pregnancy with minimal risk of viral transmission.[8]

LABORATORY ASPECTS

The risk of contamination of staff is extremely low but it is essential to evaluate each stage in these complex technologies very carefully to ensure their safety as much as possible. Nosocomial contamination between patients has been described both for the HIV virus and in assisted reproductive techniques for the HCV and HBV. An IVF laboratory is a complex structure where everything is planned to promote adequate conditions for cell survival and culture, a condition also favorable for viruses and bacteria. Special attention should be given to motivation and training of the fertility clinic staff who are not accustomed to handle infected patients (especially HIV positive patients) and may express anxiety. Some can even react aggressively as an expression of fear for their own safety.[1] The use of universal precautions in the processing of samples will minimize the chance of transmission of HIV to the laboratory personnel. This applies to the handling of all samples: semen, sperm preparations, follicular fluid at the time of egg retrieval, and human oocytes and embryos. A number of quality-control and infection-control techniques are used today in embryology and andrology laboratories to prevent cross-contamination between samples during processing. *In vitro* fertil-ization programs may choose to group infected samples together (e.g. before scheduled laboratory shut-downs) to decrease the chance of cross-contamination from infected to uninfected samples. The laboratory can then be cleaned during the shut-down time, before processing of uncontaminated samples begins. Other preventive measures may include the use of separate freezers for storing cryopreserved samples from infected and uninfected patients. Because virus cross-contamination has been reported between samples stored in liquid nitrogen, storing samples (e.g. sperm or embryos) from infected patients in liquid nitrogen vapor may provide an added margin of safety and help prevent cross-contamination.[9]

SCREENING FOR SEROPOSITIVE MALE PARTNERS

Screening is must for all the patients under going ART procedure, but special screening for the infected male partner is most important as follows:[10]

i. Be under active medical surveillance by an infectious disease specialist.
ii. Have plasma HIV RNA viral counts less than 50,000 copies/mL, stable over six months (preferably undetectable).
iii. Have a $CD4^+$ count of more than 250 cells/mm^3 (preferably >400).
iv. Have no evidence of AIDS or worsening infection.
v. If not well controlled, taking highly active antiretroviral therapy.
vi. Undergo semen analysis with total motile sperm of at least 1 million.
vii. Undergo blood screening for syphilis, hepatitis B and hepatitis C.

SPERM SEPARATION TECHNIQUE

The ideal technique should:

i. be quick, easy and cost-effective.
ii. isolate as much motile spermatozoa as possible.
iii. not cause sperm damage or non-physiological alterations of the separated sperm cells.
iv. eliminate dead spermatozoa and other cells, including leukocytes and bacteria.
v. eliminate toxic or bioactive substances like decapacitation factors or reactive oxygen species (ROS).
vi. allow processing of larger volumes of ejaculates.

Since none of the methods available meets all these requirements, a variety of sperm separation techniques is mandatory in clinical practice to obtain an optimal yield of functionally competent spermatozoa for insemination purposes.[11] The colloidal silica density gradients must be considered the most appropriate and generally applicable clinical sperm preparation technique. Processed semen that utilizes density-gradient centrifugation and 'swim-up' techniques is routinely performed by laboratories prior to either IUI or IVF, and these have become popular options for serodiscordant couples seeking to safely become parents. After being diluted in medium, unfractionated semen samples are filtered to remove any fibers, microcalculus and mucinous debris. The remaining sperm sediment is then layered onto a linear gradient of solution and pelleted by centrifugation. The spermatozoa pellet, now separated from seminal plasma and seminal nonspermatozoa cells, is washed, overlaid with medium and incubated for 20 to 30 minutes to allow motile spermatozoa to swim-up. The resulting supernatant containing motile spermatozoa is then collected. This semen-processing method, which effectively both segregates HIV from the cellular fraction (lymphocytes) and free virus from the sperm fraction, is termed 'sperm washing', and is still commonly used today with continued success. Although IUI and IVF-ICSI demonstrated great success in terms of minimizing risk of seroconversion, IUI may be less effective compared with IVF in terms of pregnancy outcome results.[10] It is possible to collect spermatozoa with evidence of the absence of HIV-1 RNA and proviral DNA from semen of HIV-infected males. Whatever method is used for assisted reproductive technique and for removal of HIV from semen to reduce the risk of secondary transmission, it is essential to confirm the absence of HIV-1 RNA and proviral DNA in the sperm preparation used for the assisted reproductive technique with the most sensitive tests possible. Therefore, when the specimen is being prepared for IUI or IVF-ICSI, after the washing procedure, an aliquot of washed semen (~100 µL) is commonly tested using PCR for detectable HIV-RNA prior to the sample being used for treatment.[12] In many labs, it is mandatory for couples to freeze a washed negative sample as a backup in case residual HIV is found in a post-wash sample that would otherwise necessitate cycle cancelation. Nicopoullos JD et al. (2010), have recently adopted a new laboratory protocol that uses two instead of three wash cycles after density-gradient centrifugation, and they only require the swim-up method for IUI cycles for male patients not receiving highly active antiretroviral therapy (HAART), with detectable viral loads or with semen samples with significant debris. With the new laboratory protocol, they have noted a significantly higher proportion of total motile sperm available for IUI.[13]

SEMEN PREPARATION FROM INFECTED SAMPLE

Double Density Gradient Centrifugation with Swim-up

Most protocols recommend the use of antiretroviral therapies to reduce viral load, subsequent testing of sperm samples for residual viral HIV-RNA and DNA using sensitive polymerase chain reaction (PCR) techniques, and the preparation of cleared samples for clinical use via density gradient centrifugation.

Colloidal silica density gradient in combination with swim-up has also been reported to reduce the viral load from samples carrying an infectious agent such as HIV. These procedures were developed to separate virus infected nonsperm cells and seminal plasma (in the density gradient supernatant) from HIV free, motile spermatozoa in the swim-up (from the density gradient pellet). Density gradient centrifugation provides for a substantial separation of progressively motile, high quality spermatozoa by virtue of their enhanced velocity and relatively high density[14] and at the same time produces high quality samples that are essentially free from microbial or other contaminants.[15] It has been demonstrated that the density gradient system keep lipid peroxidation of spermatozoa low by separating most of the ROS-producing cells from the normal and functional cells and that spermatozoa prepared by this approach have an enhanced capacity for fertilization.[16]

The best density gradient substance and most widely used in clinical application has been percoll.[17] However, a few years ago serious concern was expressed because of PVP component and endotoxin level of percoll, a colloidal polyvinyl pyrolidone (PVP)-coated silica particle preparation. This is why percoll should definitely not be used any more for human gametes. Other colloidal gradients which are assumed to be less harmful contain silica particles coated with silane instead of PVP.

EQUIPMENT AND DISPOSABLES

1. Laminar flow hood
2. Microscope
3. 37°C incubator
4. Centrifuge machine

5. Test tube warmer
6. Makler chamber
7. Wide mouth collection jar
8. Permanent marker pen for labeling
9. Pipettor 2 to 200 μL (Tarson) and microtips (2–200 Eppendorf)
10. Serological pipette 1, 5, 10 mL (Falcon)
11. Transfer pipettes 3 mL (Falcon)
12. Polystyrene conical tube 15 mL (Falcon)
13. Round bottom tube 14 mL (Falcon)
14. Round bottom tube 5 mL (Falcon)
15. Powder free sterile gloves
16. Tissue paper.

MEDIUM FOR SPERM PREPARATION

1. Colloidal density gradient kit
   Upper layer: 40%
   Lower layer: 80%
2. Sperm buffered medium
3. Sperm washing medium.

PROCEDURE

All the material must be labeled with the name of patient and laboratory ID number.

1. Prepare sufficient tubes for each patient:
   a. Using a sterile Pasteur pipette dispense 1.0 mL of 40% (upper layer) into a 15 mL conical tube.
   b. Then, carefully add 1.0 mL of 80% (lower layer) underneath the upper layer. A clear interface should be visible between the two layers.
2. Now, carefully overlay 1.0 mL liquefied semen (fresh or thawed) or sperm suspension directly on top of gradient. Ensure gradients are at room temperature before over layering. Cap the tube tightly.
3. Centrifuge at 300 to 400 g for 15 to 30 minutes in a swing out rotor with sealed buckets. More than one tube per semen sample may be used, if necessary.
4. Gently remove all most of the supernatant from the sperm pellet.
5. Gently aspirate the remaining solution and pellet and transfer to a fresh conical tube containing 5 to 10 mL of medium and mix gently.
6. Avoid contact with the sides of the tube to minimize carryover of seminal plasma and debris.
7. Centrifuge at 200 to 300 g for 5 to 10 minutes.
8. Repeat the washing procedure (4–7 steps).
9. Remove supernatant and gently overlay 0.5 to 1.0 mL medium and incubated for 20 to 30 minutes to allow motile spermatozoa to swim-up.
10. The resulting supernatant containing motile spermatozoa is then collected.

11. Assess sperm quality in the final sample and calculate volume required for insemination. *Note:* Send an aliquot of washed semen (~100 μL) for PCR for HIV-RNA before the insemination procedure.

REFERENCES

1. Yvon Englert, Benoit Lesage, Jean-Paul Van Vooren, Corinne Liesnard, Isabelle Place, Anne-Sophie Vannin, et al. Medically assisted reproduction in the presence of chronic viral diseases. Human Reproduction Update. 2004;10(2):149-62.
2. Raquel Loja Vitorino, Beatriz Gilda Grinsztejn, Carlos Augusto Ferreira de Andrade, Yara Hahr Marques Hökerberg, Claudia Teresa Vieira de Souza, Ruth Khalili Friedman, et al. Fertility and Sterility. 2011;95(5):1684-90.
3. Luca Mencaglia, Patrizia Falcone, Giuseppe Mario Lentini, Sabina Consigli, Manuela Pisoni, Vincenzo Lofiego, et al. ICSI for treatment of human immunodeficiency virus and hepatitis C virus-serodiscordant couples with infected male partner. Human Reproduction. 2005;20(8):2242-6.
4. Semprini AE, Persico T, Thlers T, Oneta M, Tuveri R, Serafini P, et al. Absence of hepatitis C virus and detection of hepatitis G virus/GB virus C RNA sequences in the semen of infected men. J Infect Dis. 1998;177:848-54.
5. Levy R, Tardy JC, Bourlet T, Cordonier H, Mion F, Lornage J, et al. Transmission risk of hepatitis C virus in assisted reproductive techniques. Hum Reprod. 2000;15:810-6.
6. Semprini AE, Vucetich AG, Oneta M, Rezek E, Chelo E, Hall V. Sperm washing and ICSI for men with HIV infection wishing for a child. Fertil Steril. 2001;76:S246.
7. Ethics Committee of the American Society for Re-productive Medicine. Human immunodeficiency virus and infertility treatment. Fertil Steril. 2004;82(Suppl 1):S228-31.
8. Raquel Loja Vitorino, Beatriz Gilda Grinsztejn, Carlos Augusto Ferreira de Andrade, Yara Hahr Marques Hökerberg, Claudia Teresa Vieira de Souza, Ruth Khalili Friedman, et al. Systematic review of the effectiveness and safety of assisted reproduction techniques in couples serodiscordant for human immunodeficiency virus where the man is positive. Fertility and Sterility. 2011;95(5): 1684-90.
9. Anthony Al-Khan, Jose Colon, Vidya Palta, Arlene Bardeguez. Assisted Reproductive Technology for Men and Women Infected with Human Immunodeficiency Virus Type 1 Clinical Infectious Diseases. 2003;36:195-200.
10. Brian A Levine, Sahadat K Nurudeen, Jennifer T Gosselin, Mark V Sauer. Addressing the Fertility needs of HIV-seropositive Males. Future Virology. 2011;6(3):299-306.
11. Ralf R Henkel, Wolf-Bernhard Schill. Sperm preparation for ART Reproductive Biology and Endocrinology. 2003;1:108.
12. Shingo Kato, Hideji Hanabusa, Satoru Kaneko, Koichi Takakuwa, Mina Suzuki, Naoaki Kuji, et al. Complete removal of HIV-1 RNA and proviral DNA from semen by the swim-up method: assisted reproduction technique using spermatozoa free from HIV-1: AIDS. 2006;20:00-00.
13. Nicopoullos JD, Almeida P, Vourliotis M, Gilling-Smith C. A decade of the United Kingdom sperm-washing program: untangling the transatlantic divide. Fertil Steril. 2010;94(6):2458-61.
14. Lessley BA, Garner DL. Isolation of motile spermatozoa by density gradient ceutifugation in percoll. Gamete Res. 1983;7:49-54.
15. Bolton VN, Warren RE, Braude PR. Removal of Bacterial contaminants from semen for *in vitro* fertilization or Artificial Insemination by the use of buoyant density centrifugation. Fertil Steril. 1986;46:1128-32.
16. Jaroudi KA, Carver-Ward JA, Hamilton CJCM, Siek UV, Sheth KV. Percoll Semen preparation enhances human ooctye fertilization in male factor intertility as shown by a randomized crossover study. Human Reprod. 1993;8:1438-42.
17. Gorus FK, Pipeleers DG. A rapid method for the fractionation of Human spermatozoa according to their progressive motility. Fertil Steril. 1981;35:662-5.

Ashok Agarwal

8 Oxidative Stress Tests

INTRODUCTION

Infertility is a problem with a large magnitude. Free oxygen radicals and other reactive oxygen species (ROS) affect both male and female gametes. ROS influence spermatozoa and oocytes as well as their local environments. Excessive production of ROS results in oxidative stress. Oxidative stress, in turn, affects spermatozoa quality, fertilization, early embryo development and implantation and ultimately, pregnancy rates. Oxidative stress affects both natural and assisted fertility. Therefore, understanding how ROS are produced and how they affect various functions is important. Also important is the ability to accurately measure them and establish reference values, which may help in identifying the possible causes leading to poor fertilization and subsequent stages of implantation and pregnancy. This will also be necessary to develop strategies that will help reduce oxidative stress especially during assisted reproductive techniques. This chapter aims to better our understanding on what free radicals are, their importance and how they can be measured accurately in a laboratory setting.

What are Free Radicals?

Free radicals are a group of highly reactive chemical molecules that have one or more unpaired electrons and can oxidatively modify biomolecules that they encounter. This causes them to react almost instantly with any substance in their vicinity.[1] Generally, free radicals attack the nearest stable molecule, "stealing" its electron. When the "attacked" molecule loses its electron, it becomes a free radical itself, beginning a chain reaction. Once the process is started, it can cascade and ultimately lead to the disrupting of living cells.

Types of Free Radicals

ROS represent a broad category of molecules that indicate the collection of radicals and non-radical oxygen derivatives. In addition, there is another class of free radicals that are nitrogen derived called reactive nitrogen species (RNS).[2] These reactive species are readily converted into reactive non-radical species by enzymatic or non-enzymatic chemical reactions that in turn can give rise to new radicals (Table 8.1).

Table 8.1. Examples of free radicals

Reactive oxygen species	*Reactive nitrogen species*
• Superoxide anion (O_2)	Nitric oxide (NO)
• Hydrogen peroxide (H_2O_2)	Nitric dioxide (NO_2)
• Hydroxyl radical (OH)	Peroxynitrite ($ONOO^-$)

Generation of Free Radicals in the Seminal Ejaculate

Human semen consists of different types of cells such as mature and immature spermatozoa, round cells from different stages of the spermatogenic process, leukocytes and epithelial cells. Of these, leukocytes (neutrophils and macrophages) and immature spermatozoa are the two main sources of ROS.[3,4]

Reactive oxygen species are produced by spermatozoa when a defect occurs during spermatogenesis that results in the retention of cytoplasmic droplets.[5] The retention of excess residual cytoplasm is the link between poor sperm quality and elevated ROS. Spermatozoa carrying cytoplasmic droplets are thought to be immature and functionally defective.[6] There is a strong positive correlation between immature spermatozoa and ROS production, which in turn is negatively correlated with sperm quality. Furthermore, as the concentration of immature spermatozoa in the human ejaculate increases, so does the concentration of mature spermatozoa with damaged DNA.[7]

Peroxidase-positive leukocytes are believed to be the main source of ROS in semen. Reports suggest that positive peroxidase staining may be an accurate indicator of excessive ROS even at concentrations below the World Health Organization (WHO) cutoff value for leukocytospermia (concentration $> 1 \times 10^6$ peroxidase positive leukocytes/mL semen).[8,9] The extent of damage caused by ROS resulting in sperm cell dysfunction depends on the nature, amount and duration of ROS exposure in addition to temperature, oxygen tension, concentration of ions, proteins and ROS scavengers.[10]

What is Oxidative Stress?

Oxidative stress (OS) is the term applied when oxidants outnumber antioxidants.[11] It is a common condition caused by biological systems in aerobic conditions such that antioxidants cannot scavenge the free radicals. This causes an excessive generation of ROS, which damages cells, tissues and organs.[12,13] Evidence suggests that OS induced by ROS such as superoxide anion (O_2^-), hydroxyl radicals (OH^-) and a range of lipid peroxyl radicals produced in vascular cells is involved in the pathogenesis of a wide range of diseases of the reproductive system such as varicocele, endometriosis and infection.[4,14]

Measurement of Free Radicals

Measurement of ROS is a helpful tool in the initial evaluation and follow-up of infertile male patients because high levels of OS seem to be strongly correlated with reduced fertility.[11] Numerous assays for ROS measurement have been introduced recently[14] (Table 8.2).

Table 8.2: Currently available tests for detection of reactive oxygen species (direct) or their oxidized products (indirect)

Assay	*Probe*	*Extracellular/Intracellular*
Direct Measurement		
Tetrazolium nitroblue[15]	Ferricytochrome C	Extracellular
Chemiluminescence[16,17]	Luminol	Both
	Lucigenin	Extracellular
Indirect Measurement		
Lipid peroxidation levels[15,18]	Thiobarbituric acid reactive substances	Measures oxidized component in the body fluids
Antioxidants, micronutrients, vitamins[19,20]	High-performance liquid chromatography	Serum and seminal plasma
Ascorbate[21]	High-performance liquid chromatography	Seminal plasma
Antioxidants enzymes[22-24]	Superoxide dismutase	Seminal plasma
	Catalase	Seminal plasma
	Glutathione peroxidase	Spermatozoa
	Glutathione reductase	Spermatozoa
Chemokines[22,25]	ELISA	Seminal plasma
Antioxidant-prooxidant status	Total antioxidant capacity	Low molecular chain breaking antioxidants

The chemiluminescence method is the most commonly used technique for measuring ROS produced by spermatozoa.[26] This assay quantifies both intracellular and extracellular ROS. Depending on the probe used, this method can differentiate between the production of superoxide and hydrogen peroxide by spermatozoa.

Luminometers

A variety of luminometers can be used to measure the light intensity resulting from the chemiluminescence reaction. Although, all luminometers utilize photomultiplier tubes to detect photons, they differ in the processing of signal input. Two different processing designs are presently found in luminometers. Photon counting luminometers count individual photons whereas direct current luminometers measure electric current that is maintained by, and is proportional to, the photon flux passing through the photomultiplier tube. The results are expressed as relative units (RLU), counted photons pre minute (cpm) or milivolts/sec.

Various models of luminometers are available and they differ in price, design and features (Table 8.3). When comparing models, it is important to check their coefficient of variation and the lower limit of detection. Three types of luminometers are commercially available. Single/double tube luminometers are inexpensive and can measure only one or two samples at a given time. These are suitable for small research laboratories. Multiple tube luminometers are more expensive because they can measure multiple samples at one time. These are suitable

Table 8.3: Some commercially available luminometer models: price and manufacturers[26]

Model	*Type*	*Sensitivity and dynamic range*	*Price (US $)*	*Manufacturer*
TD 20/20*	Single tube	0.1 fg luciferase, >5 orders	5,250	Turner biosystems Inc., Sunnyvale, CA, USA
FB-12*	Single tube	1000 molecules of luciferase, 6 orders	5,350	Zylux Corporation, Oak Ridge, TN, USA
Traithler	Single tube	1-10 pg ATP, 7 orders	6,000	Bioscan, Washington, DC, USA
Zylux FB 15*	Single tube	1000 molecules of luciferase, >6 orders	7,450	Bio-World, Dublin, OH, USA
Optocomp-2*	Multiple tube	0.1 pg ATP, 6 orders	14,160	MGM Instruments, Inc., Hamden, CT, USA
Autolumat LB 953**	Multiple tube	5 amol of ATP, 6 orders	18,000	Berthold Technologies, Oak Ridge, TN, USA
MicroLumi XS*	Microplate	0.1 fg luciferase, >6 orders	9,000	Harta Instruments, Gaithersburg, MD, USA
Luminoskan*	Microplate	<0.5 fmol ATP, 6 orders	20,000	GMI, Inc., Albertville, MN, USA

ATP = adenosine 5' triphosphate.

* Instrument offers the option of direct data transfer to personal computer.

** Instrument has ability to measure in a range of 1-10^6 counts without saturation. Beyond this range the instrument has a linear response to the signal input.

for centers that are engaged in large scale research that measure ROS in samples by chemiluminescence very frequently. Plate luminometers can analyze multiple samples on a single plate. Each plate is disposable and is relatively inexpensive (approximately $5 each). However, the entire plate must be disposed of, even when measuring luminescence for a single sample. These luminometers are therefore more suitable for commercial entities and core research laboratories.[26]

Multiple factors affect chemiluminescent reactions. These include the concentration of reaction mixture, sample volume, temperature control and background luminescence. The person who operates these instruments should be familiar with these factors, which will enable them to obtain consistently accurate results.[27] Our center currently uses the LB953 luminometer (Model: LKB 953, Wallac Inc., Gaithersburg, MD), which is a photoncounting instrument that covers a spectral range from 390 to 620 nm.

Chemiluminescence Measurement

Equipment and Material

i. Disposable polystyrene tubes with caps (15 mL)
ii. Eppendorf pipets (5 μL, 10 μL)

iii. Serological Pipets (1 mL, 2 mL, 10 mL)
iv. Desk top centrifuge
v. Disposable MicroCell Slides
vi. Dimethyl Sulfoxide (DMSO; Catalog # D8779, Sigma Chemical Co. , St. Louis, MO)
vii. Luminol (5-amino-2,3 dihydro-1,4 phthalazinedione; Catalog # A8511, Sigma Chemical Co., St. Louis, MO)
viii. Polystyrene Round bottom tubes (6 mL)
ix. Luminometer (Model: LKB 953, Wallac Inc., Gaithersburg, MD)
x. Dulbecco's Phosphate Buffered Saline Solution 1X (PBS-1X; Catalog #9235, Irvine Scientific, Santa Ana, CA)

Reagent Preparation

a. *Stock Luminol (100 mM):* Weigh 177.09 mg of luminol and add it to 10 mL of DMSO solution in a polystyrene tube. The tube must be covered in aluminium foil due to the light sensitivity of the luminol. It can be stored at room temperature in the dark until the expiration date.
b. *Working Luminol (5 mM):* Mix 20 μL luminol stock solution with 380 μL DMSO in a foil-covered polystyrene tube. This must be done prior to every use. Store at room temperature in the dark until needed.
c. *DMSO Solution:* Provided ready to use. Store at room temperature until the expiration date.

Specimen Preparation and ROS Measurement

Allow the semen sample to undergo liquefaction in a 37°C incubator for 20 minutes. Next, record the initial characteristics such as volume, pH and color and manually verify sperm count and motility. After liquefaction, process the semen specimens for ROS measurement as briefly described:[28]

1. Samples are centrifuged at 300x g for 7 minutes, and the seminal plasma is removed.
2. The sperm pellet is suspended in 3 mL of Dulbecco's PBS solution (Irvine Scientific, Santa Ana, CA) and washed again at 300x g for 7 minutes.
3. The sperm concentration is adjusted to 20×10^6/mL before ROS measurement. ROS formation is measured by a chemiluminescence assay using 5 μL of luminol (5 mM, 5-amino-2, 3-dihydro-1, 4-phthalazinedione, Sigma Chemical Company, St Louis, MO).
4. Chemiluminescence is measured in the integration mode using a LB 953 luminometer (Model: LKB 953, Wallac Inc., Gaithersburg, MD) at 37°C for 15 minutes after the luminol is added. Reactive oxygen species production is expressed as counted photons per minute (cpm)/20×10^6 sperm.

Types of Samples for ROS Measurement

ROS measurement can be performed in various types of samples such as:

1. Neat or unprocessed, whole seminal ejaculate.[29]

2. *Processed sample:* Seminal plasma is removed by washing and the sample is resuspended in the culture media.[26] Measurement is done after liquefied semen specimens are centrifuged at x 300 g for 7 minutes and seminal plasma is removed. The sperm pellet is washed and resuspended to 1 mL volume in PBS. With this method the seminal plasma and other dissolved components are removed. However, all the cellular components such as debris, round cells, white blood cells and leukocytes are still present in the sample.
3. *Sperm preparation by the swim-up procedure:* After liquefaction, an aliquot of specimen is mixed with sperm wash media (Sage BioPharma, Bedminster, NJ) using a sterile Pasteur pipette. It is centrifuged at x 330 g for 10 minutes. The supernatant is carefully aspirated and the pellet resuspended in 3 mL of fresh sperm wash media. The resuspended sample is carefully transferred in equal parts to two 15 mL sterile round-bottom test tubes and centrifuged at x 330 g for 5 minutes. Motile sperm are allowed to swim up during the incubation of test tubes at a 45° angle in 5% CO_2 at 37°C for 1 hour. Supernatant is aspirated into a clean test tube and centrifuged at x 330 g for 7 minutes. The final supernatant is aspirated and the sperm pellet resuspended in 0.5 mL of sperm wash media. The final volume is measured, and the semen analysis is performed on an aliquot of the sample.[30]
4. *Sperm preparation by density gradients:* With this method, a double density gradient (40% 'Upper phase' and 80% 'Lower phase') is used.[30] Both the density gradient and the sperm wash media is brought to 37°C or room temperature. Using a sterile pipette, 2.0 mL of the "lower phase" is transferred into a 15 mL conical centrifuge tube. Using a new sterile pipette, 2.0 mL of the "upper layer" is carefully placed on the top of the lower layer. The liquefied semen sample (1-2 mL) is placed on top of the upper layer, and the tube is centrifuged for 20 minutes at 330x g. The upper and lower layers are carefully aspirated without disturbing the pellet. Using a transfer pipette, 2 to 3 mL of sperm wash media (Sage BioPharma, Bedminster, NJ) is added, and the resuspended pellet is centrifuged for 7 minutes at 330x g. The supernatant is removed, and the pellet is suspended in 1.0 mL of sperm wash media. Sperm count, motility and ROS levels are measured in the recovered fractions.

ROS Measurement by Luminometer

After turning on the luminometer, label seven 6 mL tubes and add reagents as shown in Table 8.4. This procedure must occur in subdued light.

Enter the Information in the Luminometer

a. *Protocol:* Enter the patient information, number of samples, single measuring time and data points measured in the integrated mode. Generally, the measurement time is 15 minutes.
b. *Measurement:* Here, the file name must be entered. Verify the information is accurate.

Run the assay, and when measurement is complete, add the details of each tube in the comments section. Go to "evaluation" and check the results, which can also be printed.

Table 8.4: Steps showing the assay protocol for measuring ROS

No.	*Labeled tube*	*PBS vol*.*	*Specimen vol.*	*Luminol (5 mM)*
1.	Blank	400 μL	—	
2.	Control 1	400 μL	—	10 μL
3.	Control 1	400 μL	—	10 μL
4.	Patient 1	—	400 μL	10 μL
5.	Patient 1	—	400 μL	10 μL
6.	Patient 2	—	400 μL	10 μL
7.	Patient 2	—	400 μL	10 μL

Note: To avoid contamination, change pipette tips after each addition.
*Blank and control tubes should ideally contain filtered seminal plasma. However, we found no differences in ROS levels between filtered seminal plasma and PBS. For convenience, PBS can be used instead of filtered seminal plasma.

Calculation of ROS Results

a. Calculate the average of the control tubes.
b. Calculate the average of each set of patient sample tubes. Subtract the control value from the test value.
c. The results must be expressed as $x10^6$ counted photons per minute (cpm).
d. Next, the results must be expressed as cpm /20 million sperm. To calculate this, plug in the actual sperm concentration and multiply by the appropriate factor.

For example:

Sperm count = 8.5×10^6 sperm/mL and ROS levels are 0.2×10^6 cpm
To express this per 20×10^6 sperm/mL

$$\frac{0.2 \times 20}{8.5} = 0.47 \times 10^6 \text{ cpm}/ 20 \times 10^6 \text{ sperm}$$

The cutoff values for abnormal ROS levels depend on the type of sample: Values $> 0.2 \times 10^6$ cpm/ 20 x 10^6 sperm for neat sample and $> 1 \times 10^6$ cpm/ 20×10^6 sperm for washed samples are considered to be ROS positive.

Reference Values for Abnormal ROS

Recently, measurement of ROS in neat semen has proved to be an accurate and reliable test for assessing the OS status.[29] Also, assessing ROS directly in neat semen has diagnostic and prognostic capabilities identical to that of the ROS-TAC score. This methodology accurately represents the true *in vivo* OS status of an individual and overcomes the drawbacks of earlier methods as the processing of semen may generate ROS by itself. However, sperm preparation is necessary to enhance and maintain sperm quality and function following ejaculation before it can be used for assisted reproduction.[29] Levels of ROS were significantly lower in neat semen than in washed spermatozoa. However, ROS levels in neat semen showed a strong positive correlation with ROS levels in washed semen.[31,32] The measurement of ROS levels for fertile donors with normal semen parameters was 1.5×10^4 cpm/20 million sperm/mL. Using this cutoff, infertile men can be classified as either OS positive ($>1.5 \times 10^4$ cpm/20 million sperm/mL) or OS-negative ($<1.5 \times 10^4$ cpm/20 million sperm/mL), irrespective of their clinical diagnosis or results of standard semen analysis.[32]

Probes for Extracellular and Intracellular ROS Measurement

Two probes may be used with the chemiluminescence assay: luminol and lucigenin. A luminol-mediated chemiluminescence signal in spermatozoa occurs when luminol oxidizes at the acrosomal level. Luminol reacts with a variety of ROS and allows both intracellular and extracellular ROS to be measured. Lucigenin, however, yields a chemiluminescence that is more specific for superoxide anions released extracellularly.[17,33]

The luminol assay is more advantageous for a number of reasons. It can measure H_2O_2, $O_2^{\bullet-}$, and $OH^{\bullet-}$ levels, although it cannot distinguish these oxidants from one another.[14] It can also measure the global level of ROS under physiological conditions, and it is easy to use. In addition, the assay can measure both extracellular and intracellular ROS, which means it has a high sensitivity.[14] Multiple studies have correlated high chemiluminescent signals using luminol as a probe with adverse effects on sperm function. The assay can be sensitized by adding horseradish peroxidase to the sperm suspension, thereby increasing the spontaneous luminescence levels commonly observed in healthy semen samples.[33]

SUMMARY

ROS are necessary for various physiological functions but an imbalance in favor of ROS results in OS. Reactive oxygen species can be measured in a variety of fluids from both males and females and are involved in the pathophysiology of infertility. Various techniques as well as instruments are available for accurately measuring ROS. Supplementation with appropriate antioxidants may be beneficial in reducing the harmful effects of ROS.

REFERENCES

1. Warren JS, Johnson KJ, Ward PA. Oxygen radicals in cell injury and cell death. Pathol Immunopathol Res. 1987;6:301-15.
2. Sikka SC. Relative impact of oxidative stress on male reproductive function. Curr Med Chem. 2001;8:851-62.
3. Aitken RJ, West KM. Analysis of the relationship between reactive oxygen species production and leucocyte infiltration in fractions of human semen separated on Percoll gradients. Int J Androl. 1990;13:433-51.
4. Hendin BN, Kolettis PN, Sharma RK, Thomas AJ Jr., Agarwal A. Varicocele is associated with elevated spermatozoal reactive oxygen species production and diminished seminal plasma antioxidant capacity. J Urol. 1999;161:1831-4.
5. Gomez E, Buckingham DW, Brindle J, Lanzafame F, Irvine DS, Aitken RJ. Development of an image analysis system to monitor the retention of residual cytoplasm by human spermatozoa: correlation with biochemical markers of the cytoplasmic space, oxidative stress, and sperm function. J Androl. 1996;17:276-87.

6. Huszar G, Sbracia M, Vigue L, Miller DJ, Shur BD. Sperm plasma membrane remodeling during spermiogenetic maturation in men: relationship among plasma membrane beta 1,4-galactosyltransferase, cytoplasmic creatine phosphokinase, and creatine phosphokinase isoform ratios. Biol Reprod. 1997;56:1020-4.
7. Gil-Guzman E, Ollero M, Lopez MC, Sharma RK, Alvarez JG, Thomas AJ Jr., Agarwal A. Differential production of reactive oxygen species by subsets of human spermatozoa at different stages of maturation. Hum Reprod. 2001;16:1922-30.
8. Sharma RK, Pasqualotto FF, Nelson DR, Thomas AJ Jr., Agarwal A. Relationship between seminal white blood cell counts and oxidative stress in men treated at an infertility clinic. J Androl. 2001; 22:575-83.
9. Novotny J, Oborna II, Brezinova J, Svobodova M, Hrbac J, Fingerova H. The occurrence of reactive oxygen species in the semen of males from infertile couples. Biomed Pap Med Fac Univ Palacky Olomouc Czech Repub. 2003;147:173-6.
10. Agarwal A, Saleh RA. Role of oxidants in male infertility: rationale, significance, and treatment. Urol Clin North Am. 2002;29:817-27.
11. Sharma RK, Pasqualotto FF, Nelson DR, Thomas AJ Jr., Agarwal A. The reactive oxygen species-total antioxidant capacity score is a new measure of oxidative stress to predict male infertility. Hum Reprod. 1999;14:2801-7.
12. Aitken RJ, Baker HW. Seminal leukocytes: passengers, terrorists or good samaritans? Hum Reprod. 1995;10:1736-9.
13. Pasqualotto FF, Sharma RK, Kobayashi H, Nelson DR, Thomas AJ Jr., Agarwal A. Oxidative stress in normospermic men undergoing infertility evaluation. J Androl. 2001;22:316-22.
14. Sharma RK, Agarwal A. Role of reactive oxygen species in male infertility. Urology. 1996;48:835-50.
15. Alvarez JG, Touchstone JC, Blasco L, Storey BT. Spontaneous lipid peroxidation and production of hydrogen peroxide and superoxide in human spermatozoa. Superoxide dismutase as major enzyme protectant against oxygen toxicity. J Androl. 1987;8:338-48.
16. McKinney KA, Lewis SE, Thompson W. Reactive oxygen species generation in human sperm: luminol and lucigenin chemiluminescence probes. Arch Androl. 1996;36:119-25.
17. Aitken RJ, Buckingham DW, West KM: Reactive oxygen species and human spermatozoa: analysis of the cellular mechanisms involved in luminol- and lucigenin-dependent chemiluminescence. J Cell Physiol. 1992;151:466-77.
18. Aitken RJ, Clarkson JS, Fishel S. Generation of reactive oxygen species, lipid peroxidation, and human sperm function. Biol Reprod. 1989;41:183-97.
19. Lenzi A, Picardo M, Gandini L, Lombardo F, Terminali O, Passi S, Dondero F. Glutathione treatment of dyspermia: effect on the lipoperoxidation process. Hum Reprod. 1994;9:2044-50.
20. Kessopoulou E, Powers HJ, Sharma KK, Pearson MJ, Russell JM, Cooke ID, Barratt CL. A double-blind randomized placebo cross-over controlled trial using the antioxidant vitamin E to treat reactive oxygen species associated male infertility. Fertil Steril. 1995;64:825-31.
21. Thiele JJ, Friesleben HJ, Fuchs J, Ochsendorf FR. Ascorbic acid and urate in human seminal plasma: determination and interrelationships with chemiluminescence in washed semen. Hum Reprod. 1995;10:110-5.
22. Rajasekaran M, Hellstrom WJ, Naz RK, Sikka SC. Oxidative stress and interleukins in seminal plasma during leukocytospermia. Fertil Steril. 1995;64:166-71.
23. Nissen HP, Kreysel HW. Superoxide dismutase in human semen. Klin Wochenschr. 1983;61:63-5.
24. Li TK. The glutathione and thiol content of mammalian spermatozoa and seminal plasma. Biol Reprod. 1975;12:641-6.
25. Buch JP, Kolon TF, Maulik N, Kreutzer DL, Das DK. Cytokines stimulate lipid membrane peroxidation of human sperm. Fertil Steril. 1994;62:186-8.

26. Agarwal A, Allamaneni SS, Said TM. Chemiluminescence technique for measuring reactive oxygen species. Reprod Biomed Online. 2004;9:466-8.
27. Berthold F, Herick K, Siewe RM. Luminometer design and low light detection. Methods Enzymol. 2000;305:62-87.
28. Kobayashi H, Gil-Guzman E, Mahran AM, Rakesh, Nelson DR, Thomas AJ Jr., Agarwal A. Quality control of reactive oxygen species measurement by luminol-dependent chemiluminescence assay. J Androl. 2001;22:568-74.
29. Allamaneni SS, Agarwal A, Nallella KP, Sharma RK, Thomas AJ Jr., Sikka SC. Characterization of oxidative stress status by evaluation of reactive oxygen species levels in whole semen and isolated spermatozoa. Fertil Steril. 2005;83:800-3.
30. Allamaneni SS, Agarwal A, Rama S, Ranganathan P, Sharma RK. Comparative study on density gradients and swim-up preparation techniques utilizing neat and cryopreserved spermatozoa. Asian J Androl. 2005;7:86-92.
31. Saleh RA, Agarwal A: Oxidative stress and male infertility: from research bench to clinical practice. J Androl. 2002;23:737-52.
32. Saleh RA, Agarwal A, Kandirali E, Sharma RK, Thomas AJ, Nada EA, Evenson DP, Alvarez JG. Leukocytospermia is associated with increased reactive oxygen species production by human spermatozoa. Fertil Steril. 2002;78:1215-24.
33. Aitken RJ, Buckingham D. Enhanced detection of reactive oxygen species produced by human spermatozoa with 7-dimethyl amino-naphthalin-1, 2- dicarbonic acid hydrazide. Int J Androl. 1992; 15:211-9.

9

Ashok Agarwal

TUNEL Test

INTRODUCTION

Dioxyribonucleic acid (DNA) fragmentation is a process which results from the activation of endonucleases during apoptosis. These nucleases degrade the higher order sperm chromatin structure into fragments ~30 kb and subsequently into smaller DNA pieces about ~50 kb in length. This method is used to detect fragmented DNA and utilizes a reaction catalyzed by exogenous terminal deoxynucleotidyl transferase (TdT) and is termed as 'end labeling' or TUNEL (terminal deoxynucleotidyl transferase dUTP nick end labeling) assay.

ASSAY PRINCIPLE

This single step staining methods labels DNA breaks with FITC-dUTP followed by flow cytometric analysis. TdT catalyzes a template-independent addition of bromolated deoxyuridine triphosphatase to the 3'-hydroxyl (OH) termini of double and single-stranded DNA. After incorporation, these sites are identified by flow cytometric means by staining the sperm.

SPECIMEN COLLECTION

- Following liquefaction, evaluate semen specimens for volume, sperm concentration, total cell count, motility and morphology
- Aliquot and load a 5 µL aliquot of the sample on a microcell slide chamber for manual evaluation of concentration and motility. Check the concentration of sperm in the sample. Adjust it to 2–3 × 10^6/mL
- Suspend the cells in 3.7% (w/v) paraformaldehyde prepared in phosphate buffered saline (PBS) (pH 7.4)

  Note: Fixing in paraformaldehyde is important to avoid loss of smaller fragments of DNA that are not chemically fixed prior to washing the samples.
- Place the cell suspension on ice for 30 to 60 minutes/overnight
- Centrifuge to pellet the cells at 300 g for seven minutes. Discard the supernatant and suspend the pellet in 1 mL of ice-cold 70% (v/v) ethanol at –20°C until use. Cells can be stored at –20°C several days before use.

STAINING PROTOCOL

- Resuspend the positive (6552LZ) and negative (6553LZ) control cells by swirling the vials.
- Remove 2 mL aliquots of the control cell suspensions (approximately 1×10^6 cells/mL) and place in 12×75 mm centrifuge tubes. Centrifuge the control cell suspensions for five minute at 300x g and remove the 70% (v/v) ethanol by aspiration, being careful to not disturb the cell pellet.
  Note: Use of polystyrene, and not polypropylene tubes (12×75 mm), is recommended to avoid cell build up, improve staining and/or loss of cells.
- Resuspend each tube of control and sample tubes with 1.0 mL of wash buffer (6548AZ) (blue cap) for each tube. Centrifuge as before and remove the supernatant by aspiration
- Repeat the wash buffer treatment.
  Note: Washing should be carried out by gentle mixing and not by pipetting to avoid cell loss.
- Resuspend each tube of the control cell pellets in 50 µL of the staining solution (prepared as described below).

STAINING SOLUTION (SINGLE ASSAY)

The staining solution consists of the following:

- Reaction buffer (green cap); TdT enzyme (yellow cap); FITC-dUTP (orange cap). The staining solution for a single assay is prepared by mixing the staining reagents as follows: Reaction buffer 10 µL + TdT enzyme 0.75 µL + FITC-dUTP 8.00 µL and distilled water 32.25 µL to give a total staining solution volume of 51.00 µL.
  Note: The appropriate volume of staining solution to prepare for a variable number of assays is based upon multiples of the component volumes needed for one assay. Mix only enough staining solution to complete the number of assays prepared per session. The staining solution is active for approximately 24 hours at 4°C.
- Incubate the sperm in the staining solution for 60 minutes at 37°C.
- At the end of the incubation time, add 1.0 mL of rinse buffer (6550AZ) (red cap) to each tube and centrifuge each tube at 300x g for five minutes. Remove the supernatant by aspiration.
- Repeat the cell rinsing with 1.0 mL of rinse buffer, centrifuge and remove the supernatant by aspiration.
- Resuspend the cell pellet in 0.5 mL of the PI/RNase staining buffer (6551AZ).
  Note: If the cell density is low, decrease the amount of PI/RNase staining buffer to 0.3 mL.
- Incubate the cells in the dark for 30 minutes at room temperature.
- Analyze the cells in PI/RNase solution by flow cytometry.
  Note: The cells must be analyzed within 3 hours of staining. Cells may begin to deteriorate, if left overnight before analysis. In addition to the negative and positive controls provided with the kit, it is also important to include the negative and positive sperm control samples.

Negative Control

In this, the TdT enzyme is omitted from the reaction mixture.

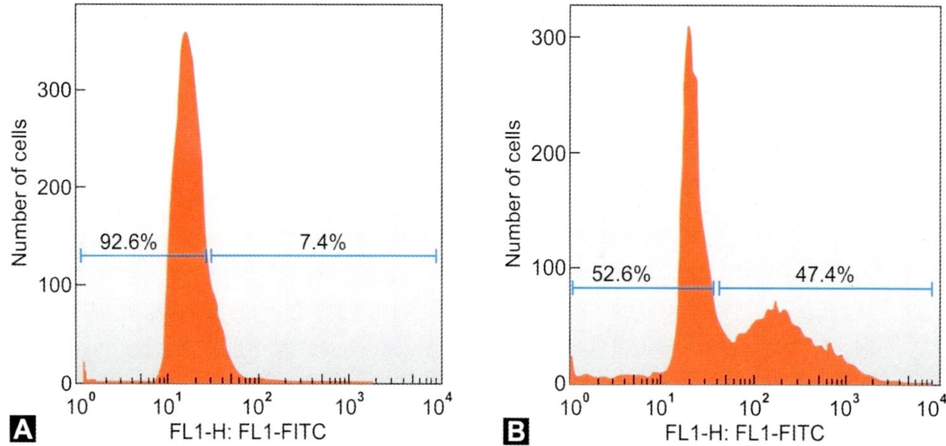

FIGURES 9.1A AND B: Representative images of sperm DNA damage as measured by the TUNEL assay. (A) Negative sample, and (B) Positive sample showing DNA damage

Positive Control

DNA damage is induced by adding 100 µL of DNase I (1 mg/mL) for 1 hour at 37°C.

FLOW CYTOMETRY

- For flow cytometry evaluation, a minimum of 10,000 events are examined for each measurement at a flow rate of about 200 events/sec on a flow cytometer (Fluorescence activated cell sorting caliber, Becton and Dickinson, San Jose, CA).
- The excitation wavelength is 488 nm supplied by an argon laser at 15 mW. Green fluorescence (480–530 nm) is measured in the FL1 channel and red fluorescence (580–630 nm) in the FL2 channel.
- Spermatozoa obtained in the plots are gated using a forward-angled light scatter and side-angled light scatter dot plot to gate out debris, aggregates and other cells different from spermatozoa.
- TUNEL positive spermatozoa in the population are measured after converting to a histogram (Figs 9.1A and B).
- The percentage of positive cells (TUNEL-positive) are calculated on a 1,023 channel scale using the appropriate flow cytometer software FlowJo Mac version 8.2.4 (FlowJo, LLC, Ashland, OR) as describe by authors earlier.[1]

FACTORS AFFECTING THE ASSAY RESULTS

Several factors are important to consider when performing this test:

- Accessibility of the DNA
- Sperm preparation

- Presence of dead cells
- Number of cells examined
- Interobserver and intraobserver as well as interassay and intra-assay variations.

REFERENCE RANGE OF SPERM DNA DAMAGE

We have recently reported the intra-assay, interassay, interobserver and intraobserver values for the TUNEL assay and reported a cut-off value (19.2%), sensitivity (64.9%) and specificity (100%) for this test.[1]

REFERENCE

1. Sharma RK, Sabanegh E, Mahfouz R, Gupta S, Thiyagarajan A, Agarwal A. TUNEL as a test for sperm DNA damage in the evaluation of male infertility. Urology. 2010;76:1380-6.

10

Rima Dada

Reactive Oxygen Species Measurement

INTRODUCTION

Reactive oxygen species (ROS) are free radicals that are derived from oxygen metabolism and contain highly reactive molecules consisting of one or more unpaired electrons. ROS could damage different parts of the spermatozoa, including both nuclear and mitochondrial DNA and thus impair sperm function. It is a well known fact that unlike somatic cells, mature spermatozoa have minimal cytoplasm. Since cytoplasm is the major source of antioxidants, scanty cytoplasm in the mature spermatozoa causes deficiency in both antioxidants and endogenous repair enzymes/factors. However, naturally the deficiency of antioxidant system is compensated by the enzymatic and non-enzymatic components of seminal fluid. Under physiological conditions, spermatozoa produce small amounts of ROS needed for capacitation, acrosome reaction and fertilization however, under pathological conditions the generated ROS overwhelms the antioxidant capacity of the seminal fluid and thus establishes oxidative stress. Therefore, it is necessary to analyze the ROS levels in the semen of men with idiopathic infertility. It has been documented that infertile men with normal and abnormal semen parameters have raised ROS levels. This indicates that ROS levels as an independent parameter should be evaluated in all infertile cases.

METHODOLOGY

Levels of ROS can be measured by a probe called luminol using chemiluminescence assay. Luminol is an extremely sensitive oxidizable substrate which reacts with a variety of ROS at neutral pH that results in production of a light signal which is then converted to electrical signal (photon) by a instrument and the free radicals produced by the instrument is measured in an integrated mode for 15 min and expressed as relative light unit per minute (RLU/min) per 20×10^6.

Sample Collection

- Obtain semen samples in a sterile plastic container from the subject after four days of sexual abstinence.
- Name of the patient and date of sample collection will be recorded in a container.

Sample Analysis

- Allow the sample to liquefy at 37°C and perform standard semen analysis as per WHO, 2010 guidelines.
- After liquefaction, note the physical characteristics such as viscosity, pH, color and odor.
- Place 10 µL of sample in a microscope slide, gently place the coverslip over the sample and observe for concentration and motility.
- Aliquot 400 µL of neat semen for ROS measurement.
- Aliquot 400 µL of neat semen for washed ROS measurement.

Instrument Setup

- Switch on the computer.
- Switch on the luminometer and connect it to the computer.
- Run FB12 sirius software and click the start icon to run after placing the sample.

Preparation of Tubes

- Prepare tubes for (1) blank, (2) positive control, (3) for an internal negative control, (4) for patient (Neat, washed semen).
- Measure the ROS levels by luminol dependent chemiluminescence assay by using single detector luminometer (Sirius, Berthold Detection Systems GmbH, Pforzheim, Germany) in the integrated mode for 15 minutes as described below.

ROS Estimation

Blank

- For measuring the blank add 400 µL of 1x PBS (pH 7.4).
- Measure the ROS levels in an integrated mode for 15 min.

Negative Control

- For measuring the internal negative control, add 400 µL of 1x PBS (pH 7.4).
- Measure the ROS levels in an integrated mode for 15 min.
- Add 10 µL of luminol to the tube and gently tap the cuvette.
- Note the readings for 15 min.

Positive Control

- For measuring positive control, add 400 µL of 1x PBS (pH 7.4).
- Measure the ROS levels in an integrated mode for 15 min.
- Add 10 µL of H_2O_2 to the tube and gently tap the cuvette.
- Note the readings for 15 min.

Measurement of ROS in Neat Semen

- Take 400 μL of the neat semen and note the readings for 15 min.
- After completion of the above step, add 10 μL of luminol (5-amino-2,3,-dihydro-1,4-phthalazinedione; Sigma), prepared as 5 mM stock in dimethyl sulfoxide (DMSO) to 400 μL of liquefied neat semen and measure the reading for 15 min.
- Measure the samples in duplicate and take the average readings.

Measurement of ROS in Washed Semen

- Levels of ROS can be measured in washed sperm suspensions using a chemiluminescence assay.[2,4]
- With this protocol, liquefied semen is centrifuged at 300 xg for 7 minutes, and the seminal plasma is separated and stored at –80°C for measurement of TAC.
- The resulting pellet is washed with phosphate-buffered saline (1x PBS)
- Discard the supernatant and resuspend the pellet in the same 1 mL washing media at a concentration of 20×10^6 sperm/mL.
- Four-hundred microliter aliquots of the resulting cell suspensions (containing sperm and leukocytes) are used to assess basal ROS levels at an integrated mode for 15 min.
- After completion of the above step, add 10 μL of luminol (5-amino-2,3,-dihydro-1,4-phthalazinedione; Biochemika) to 400 μL of liquefied neat semen and measure the reading for 15 min.

Data Analysis

- After completion of the analysis, convert the file into excel and save with particular sample detail and close the file.
- Normalize the reading with luminol from the reading without luminol to get the original value.
- Normalize the case reading from the reading of blank.

Calculation of ROS

$$\frac{\text{ROS value obtained per min} \times 20 \times 10^6 \text{ million sperms/mL}}{\text{Sperm count in 400 μL of semen}}$$

Express it as RLU/min per 20×10^6 spermatozoa

Materials Required

- Disposable slides
- Coverslips
- Pipettes (1 mL, 10 μL)
- Centrifuge
- Microcentrifuge tubes (1.5 mL)

- Sample tube
- Luminometer (Sirius, Berthold Detection Systems GmbH, Pforzheim, Germany).

Chemicals Required

- Dimethyl sulfoxide
- Luminol
- Phosphate buffer saline.

PREPARATION OF REAGENTS AND SOLUTIONS

1. Preparation of 5 mM luminol in DMSO.
   Weigh 0.008 gm of luminol (5-amino-2,3,-dihydro-1,4-phthalazinedione; Sigma) and dissolve in 10 mL of dimethylsulfoxide solution in 15 mL falcon tube and aliquot in a separate 1.5 mL tubes cover with aluminium foil, store in a refrigerator.
2. DMSO: Ready to use.
3. Preparation of 10x PBS stock:
   - Sodium chloride (NaCl) 8 gm
   - Potassium chloride (KCl) 0.20 gm
   - Disodium hydrogen phosphate (Na_2HPO_4) 1.44 gm
   - Potassium dihydrogen phosphate (KH_2PO_4) 0.24 gm

Dissolve the above chemicals in one liter of water and adjust the pH to7.4. Autoclave and store it in refrigerator.

Note:

- Measurement of ROS should be taken in a dark room.
- Sample should be kept in incubator and processed within an hour of collection.
- Change the tip after each addition of sample and luminol.

BIBLIOGRAPHY

1. Fingerova H, Oborna I, Novotny J, Svobodova M, Brezinova J, Radova L (2009) The measurement of reactive oxygen species in human neat semen and in suspended spermatozoa: A comparison. Reprod Biol Endocrinol. 7:118. doi:1477-7827-7-118.
2. Kobayashi H, Gil-Guzman E, Mahran AM, Sharma RK, Nelson DR, Thomas AJ Jr, Agarwal A. Quality control of reactive oxygen species measurement by luminol-dependent chemiluminescence assay. J Androl. 2001;22:568-74.
3. Venkatesh S, Riyaz AM, Shamsi MB, Kumar R, Gupta NP, Mittal S, Malhotra N, Sharma RK, Agarwal A, Dada R. Clinical significance of reactive oxygen species in semen of infertile Indian men. Andrologia. 2009;41:251-6.
4. Venkatesh S, Shamsi MB, Dudeja S, Kumar R, Dada R. Reactive oxygen species measurement in neat and washed semen: Comparative analysis and its significance in male infertility assessment. Arch Gynecol Obstet.
5. WHO laboratory manual for the examination of human semen and semen-cervical mucus interaction (2010), 5 edn. Cambridge University Press, Cambridge, UK.

11

Ved Prakash

Assessment of DNA Fragmentation (Halo Test)

INTRODUCTION

Routine semen analysis, following WHO guidelines, yields valuable information concerning testicular function, and is considered the gold standard in the evaluation of male infertility although it only measures the volume of the ejaculate, sperm concentration, motility and sperm cells with normal size and shape. Several recent reports have focused on the male contribution to couples' infertility and other factors within sperm have been related to male infertility. For instance, sperm mRNA subsets are now being recognized as highly relevant in early embryo development and pregnancy outcome, despite the known capacity of the oocyte to repair some sperm defects such as DNA damage.[1]

The effect of sperm DNA fragmentation on infertility has been subject of several studies. Previously, 10 to 20% DNA fragmentation was reported in ejaculated spermatozoa. The infertile men with poor sperm motility and morphology present higher levels of DNA fragmentation than individuals with normal semen parameters. Men with normal semen parameters has also suggested to have high DNA fragmentation index (DFI), which can be one of the reasons of unexplained infertility. Therefore, it is important to evaluate DNA fragmentation in infertile men before undergoing ART procedure. Aberrant chromatin packaging during spermatogenesis, defective apoptosis before ejaculation, or excessive production of reactive oxygen species (ROS) cause DNA fragmentation in sperm cells, however, the mechanisms underlying the situation has not been clarified yet.

Controversies still present on the effects of sperm DNA damage on reproductive outcome. Some studies indicated that clinical pregnancy was affected adversely by sperm DNA damage in the cases of intracytoplasmic sperm injection (ICSI). Moreover, fertilization achieved by a sperm having fragmented DNA may cause poor embryonic development, decreased implantation and pregnancy rates, and recurrent pregnancy losses. On the contrary, some others suggested that sperm DNA damage was ineffective on fertilization, embryo quality, and pregnancy rates in cases of *in vitro* fertilization (IVF) and ICSI.

Several tests are available to measure sperm DNA fragmentation levels including TUNEL, comet assay, DNA breakage detection-fluorescence *in situ* hybridization (DBD-FISH) test, the chromomycin A3 test, SCSA test and sperm chromatin dispersion (SCD) test.[2]

These techniques are difficult to implement in andrology laboratories. Expensive instrumentation and complex protocols preclude their use in routine testing. A new improved technique to determine sperm DNA fragmentation has been established for human spermatozoa, being called the SCD test. This is a simple, fast, accurate and highly reproducible method for the analysis of sperm DNA fragmentation. It may be confidently estimated under the conventional bright-field microscope. Moreover, different degrees of DNA-nuclear damage can be detected as well as the discrimination of sperm nucleoids from other cell types. Unlike other procedures, the SCD test can be used without the requirement of complex or expensive instrumentation. However, if desired, it could be visualized with automation. Finally, laboratory technicians can easily, quickly and reliably assess the test endpoints. Therefore, the improved SCD test could allow the routine screening of sperm DNA fragmentation in the basic andrology laboratory. The halosperm is a new improved SCD test based on the principle that sperm with fragmented DNA does not produce halo of dispersed DNA loops which is characteristic of sperm with non-fragmented DNA. This new technique is commercialized as a kit under the name Halosperm. Besides its application in the semen quality assessment and infertility studies, it has been demonstrated that ionizing radiation exposure increases the frequency of spermatozoa with fragmented DNA, even for several months after the exposure. Biological dosimetry using this new parameter could be easily accomplished performing the SCD procedure.

LAB PROTOCOL

Principle of the Method[3*]

Intact unfixed sperm (fresh, frozen/unthawed, diluted samples) are immersed in an inert agarose microgel on a pretreated slide. An initial acid treatment denatures DNA in those sperm cells with fragmented DNA. Following this, the lysis solution removes most of the nuclear proteins. When absence of massive DNA breakage is present, nucleoids with large haloes of spreading DNA loops, emerging from a central core are produced. However, the nucleoids from sperm with fragmented DNA either, they do not show a dispersion halo or the halo is minimal.

Material and Equipment

1. *Kit reagents (provided with the Halosperm kit):*
   - Agarose cell support (ACS): Eppendorf tube
   - Super-coated slides (SCS); 10 units
   - Solution 1 (DA) Denaturing solution
   - Solution 2 (LS) Lysis solution
   - Solution 3 (TA) Staining solution A
   - Solution 4 (TB) Staining solution B
   - Float.
2. Bright field or fluorescence microscope
3. Fridge at 4°C
4. Incubation bath(s) at 37°C and 95–100°C
5. Plastic gloves

6. Glass coverslips (24 × 24 mm)
7. Micropipettes
8. Petri dishes or similar tray
9. Disposable pipettes
10. Distilled water
11. Ethanol at 70% and 100%
12. Microwave oven
13. Fume hood.

SPERM SAMPLE

Fresh semen samples should be collected in a sterile recipient. The sperm DNA fragmentation assay should be performed immediately once the sperm sample has been obtained or thawed after cryopreservation.

Procedure

Including the sperm sample in Agarose Microgel

1. Set solutions 1 and 2 at room temperature (22°C).
2. Dilute the sperm sample in an appropriate human sperm extender or PBS to a concentration of 15 to 20 million sperms per milliliter.
3. Place an agarose eppendorf tube (ACS) in the float and incubate in a water bath at 95 to 100°C, for 5 minutes or until the agarose is fully melted. Alternatively, use a microwave oven.
4. Transfer the agarose eppendorf tube, with the float, to a water bath at 37°C and leave it for 5 minutes until the temperature has equilibrated.
5. Transfer 50 μL of the sperm sample to the agarose tube and mix gently.
6. Place a drop of 8 μL of the cell suspension onto the centre of the well and cover with a coverslip. Press gently, avoiding air bubbles formation.
7. Slides must be held in a horizontal position throughout the entire process.
8. Place the slide on a cold surface (e.g. a metal or glass plate pre-cooled at 4°C) and transfer into the fridge at 4°C, for 5 minutes to solidify the agarose.

Processing the sperm sample

9. Take the slide out of the fridge and remove the coverslip by sliding it off gently. All the processing must be performed at room temperature (22°C).
10. Place the slide horizontally on the float into a Petri dish or similar tray.
11. Apply solution 1 on the well making sure it is fully immersed. Incubate for 7 minutes. Drain by tilting and place the slide horizontally on the top of the float.
12. Apply solution 2 on the well making sure it is fully immersed. Incubate for 20 minutes. Drain by tilting and place the slide horizontally on the top of the float.
13. Wash covering the slide for 5 minutes with abundant distilled water using a disposable pipette. Drain the water by tilting and place the slide horizontally on the top of the float.

14. Dehydrate by flooding with 70% ethanol, using a disposable pipette and incubate for 2 minutes. Drain and apply 100% ethanol for 2 minutes. Drain and allow to dry.
15. After drying, the processed slides may be kept in slide boxes at room temperature in a dry and dark place for several months.

Staining and visualization

16. Place the slide horizontally on the float inside the Petri dish.
17. Apply solution 3 on the well making sure it is fully immersed. Incubate for 6 minutes. Drain by tilting and place the slide horizontally on the top of the float.
18. Apply solution 4 on the well making sure it is fully immersed. Incubate for 7 minutes. Drain by tilting and allow to dry at room temperature.
19. Visualize under bright field microscopy. If the staining is too intense, the slide may be washed in tap water. If the staining is too weak, immerse the slide in 100% ethanol, allow to dry and repeat steps 17 and 18.

SPERM CLASSIFICATION

Score a minimum of 300 sperm per sample following the criteria:

Sperm without Fragmented DNA

- *Sperm with big halo:* Those whose halo width is similar or higher than the minor diameter of the core.
- *Sperm with medium-sized halo:* Their halo size is between those with large and with very small halo.

Sperm with Fragmented DNA

- *Sperm with small halo:* The halo width is similar or smaller than 1/3 of the minor diameter of the core.
- Sperm without halo.
- *Sperm without halo and degraded:* Those that show no halo and present a core irregularly or weakly stained.

Others: Cell nuclei, which do not correspond to sperm. One of the morphological characteristics, which distinguish them, is the absence of tail. These cells must not be included in the estimation of the frequency of sperm with fragmented DNA.

Sperm Chromatin Dispersion Patterns Observed After Staining (Fig. 11.1)

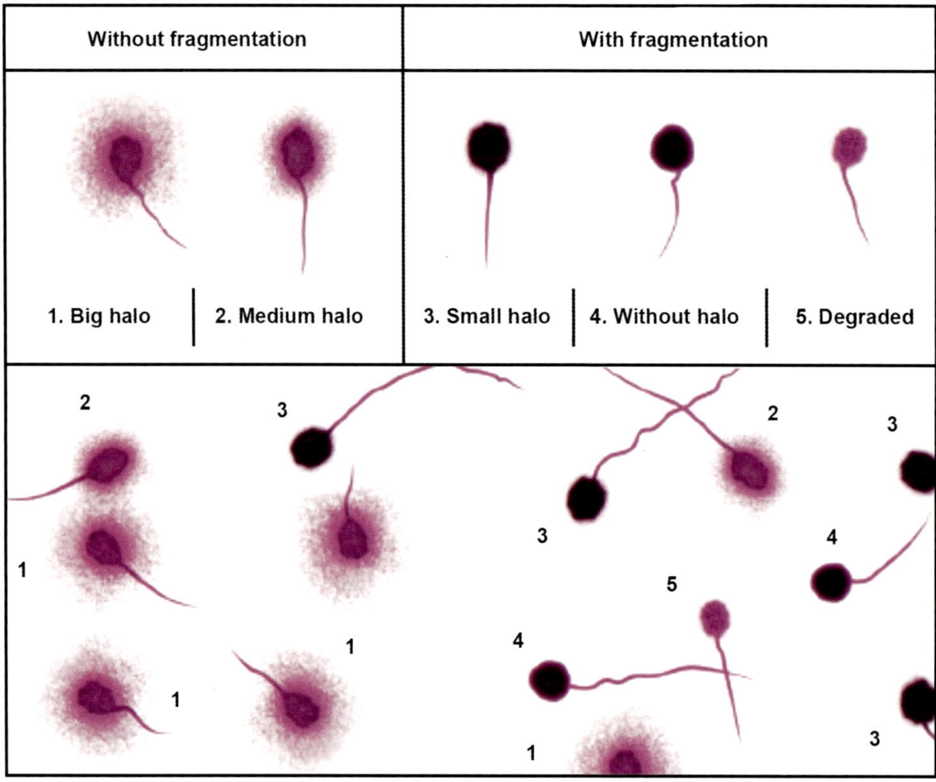

FIGURE 11.1: Sperm chromatin dispersion patterns observed after staining

$$\text{SDF (\%)} = 100 \times \frac{\text{Number of spermatozoa with fragmented DNA}}{\text{Number of spermatozoa counted}}$$

INTERPRETING THE RESULTS

Calculate the percentage of sperm with fragmented DNA. The results should be evaluated taking into account all clinical and laboratory findings related to the sperm sample.

Thresholds for frequency of DNA fragmentation index (DFI) have been suggested by Evenson et al. (J Androl. 1999;23:25-43).

DFI	*Evaluation*
<15%	Low
Between 15 and 30%	Medium
>30	High

SAFETY AND THE ENVIRONMENT

- Care should be taken to avoid contact with skin or eyes, and to prevent inhalation. LS contains Dithiothreitol and Triton X–100. Work under air removal environment and follow the manufacturer's Material Safety Data Sheet regarding safe handling.
- Do not dispose waste products into the environment.

PRECAUTIONS

- All patient samples and reagents should be treated as potentially infectious and the user must wear protective gloves, eye protection and laboratory coats when performing the test.
- The test samples should be discarded in a proper biohazard container after testing.
- Do not eat, drink or smoke in the area where specimens and kit reagents are handled.
- Do not use the kit beyond the expiration date, which appears on the package label.

REFERENCES

1. Lourdes Muriel, Marcos Meseguer, Jose Luis Fernández, Juan Alvarez, José Remohí, Antonio Pellicer and Nicolás Garrido. Value of the sperm chromatin dispersion test in predicting pregnancy outcome in intrauterine insemination: a blind prospective study. Human Reproduction 2006;21(3):738-44.
2. Seda Yýýllmaz, Asuman Demiiroglu Zergeroðllu, Elliiff Yýýllmaz, Kenan Sofuogllu, Nurii Delliikara, Pelliin Kuttllu. Effects of sperm DNA fragmentation on semen parameters and ICSI outcome determined by an Improved SCD test, Halosperm. International journal of fertility and sterility 2010;4(2):73-8.
3. *From instruction sheet provided with Halosperm kit.

12 Sperm Function Tests

MM Misro

HYPO-OSMOTIC SWELLING (HOS) TEST (PATENT FILED)[1]

Things provided: HOS solution

Storage condition: Room temperature

Apparatus required: Any ordinary microscope and micropipette (10-100 μL)

Time required: 10 minutes.

Protocol

Take 500 μL of HOS solution in a small tube. Add 50 or 100 μL (depending on high/low sperm count) of liquefied semen sample to it. Mix gently and incubate at room temperature for 5 minutes. At the end of the incubation time, one can add 50 μL of color stop solution (optional) and mix gently.

Place a small drop of the mixture on a clean glass slide and cover it with cover slip. Observe it under a microscope and count the percentage of spermatozoa with coiled tail. If the sample shows bent tail before the test, deduce the number after the test to get the actual result. Normal range: >60% with coiled tail.

Normal value: >60% bend tail (Fig. 12.1).

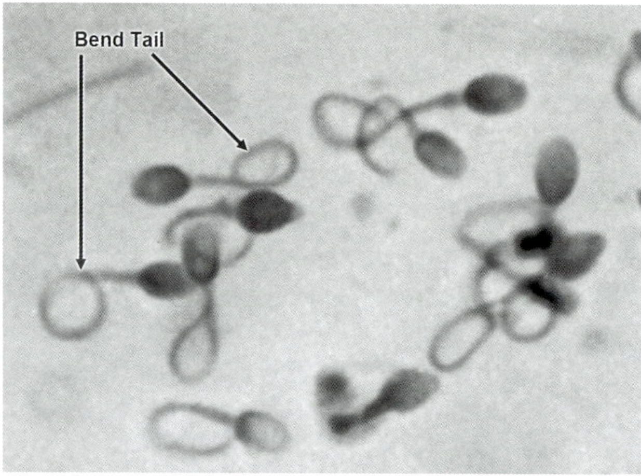

FIGURE 12.1: Bend tail (HOS)

NUCLEAR CHROMATIN DECONDENSATION TEST (PATENT FILED)

Things provided in the kit: One sachet and a color stop solution

Storage condition: 4-8°C. Once opened, the prepared solution is stable for 1 to 2 weeks when stored in refrigerator

Apparatus required: A small centrifuge, microscope, micropipette and an incubator maintained at 50°C.

Protocol

Dissolve the whole content of a sachet in 10 mL distilled water to make NCD solution. Take 500 μL of NCD solution (prewarmed at 50°C for 5 minutes) in a small tube. Add 50 to 100 μL (depending on high/low sperm count) of liquefied semen sample to it. Mix gently and incubate at 50°C temperature for 5 minutes. Stop the reaction by adding 100 μL of color stop solution. Place a small drop on a clean glass slide and cover with cover slip. Observe under the microscope and count percentage of decondensed (enlarged heads) spermatozoa. Normal range: >70% with swelled heads.

Normal value: >70% swelled head (Fig. 12.2).

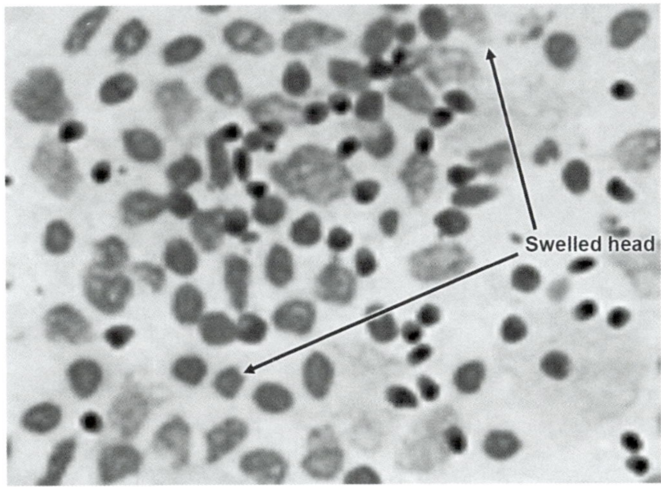

FIGURE 12.2: Swelled head (NCD)

ACROSOME STATUS AND FUNCTION (PATENT FILED)[2]

Time required: 40 minutes

Things provided in the kit: Gelatin coated slides, acrosome reaction solution

Storage condition: Room temperature

Apparatus required: Microscope, an incubator maintained at 50°C, micropipette and a moisture chamber (moisture chamber can be made using petridish lined with blotting paper and two capillary rods on which the slide rests).

Protocol

Take 500 μL of acrosome solution in a small tube. Add 50 to 100 μL (depending on high/low sperm count) of liquefied semen sample to it. Mix gently and incubate at room temperature for 5 minutes. Make a smear smoothly on a coated slide. Air dry excess liquid on the slide (care to be taken not to over dry it). Place the slide at 50°C in a moist humid chamber (the chamber should be prewarmed at 50°C) and incubate for 30 minutes. At the end of incubation time, remove the slide from the chamber, air dry it and observe it under the microscope to count percentage of spermatozoa with halos surrounding their head. Normal range: >50% spermatozoa with halos.

Normal value: >50% sperms with halos (Fig. 12.3).

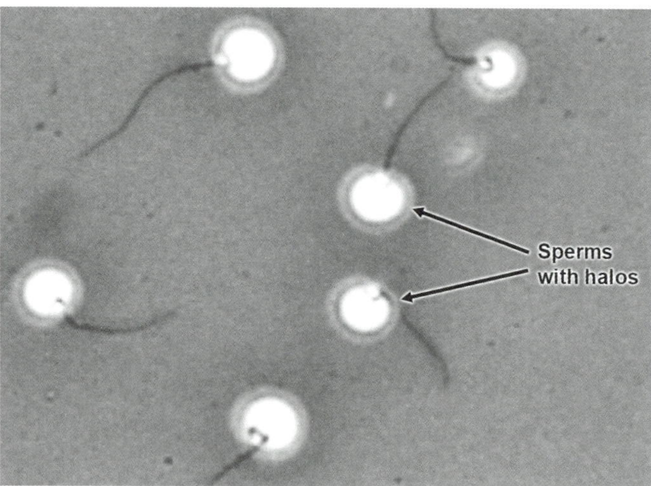

FIGURE 12.3: Sperm with halos

REFERENCES

1. Jeyendran RS, Van derVen HH, Perez-Pelaez M, Crabo BG, Zaneveld IJD. Development of an assay to assess the functional integrity of the human sperm membrane and its relationship to other semen characteristics. Journal of Reproduction and Fertility. 1984;70:219-28.
2. Gopalkrishnan, et al. Current Science. 1994;68(4)353-61.

Alex C Verghese

13 Micromanipulator Set-up and ICSI

Intracytoplasmic sperm injection (ICSI) is an *in vitro* fertilization procedure in which a single sperm is injected directly into an egg.

The technique was developed by Gianpiero Palermo around 1991 at the Vrije Universiteit Brussel, in the Center for Reproductive Medicine headed by Paul Devroey and Andre Van Steirteghem. It has been estimated that approximately 40% of sterility in couples can be attributed to male subfertility. ICSI has raised hopes that these couples can have children of their own. This method of treating predominantly male-factor patients has achieved a breakthrough, and it has established itself as the preferred method of treatment in the field of assisted reproduction.

MICROINJECTION

Microinjection is normally performed under an inverted microscope with the aid of a micromanipulator which allows for small movement under high magnification.

INTRACYTOPLASMIC SPERM INJECTION (ICSI)—PROCEDURE AND EQUIPMENT

Materials and Methods

Devices

- Inverted microscope equipped with Hoffmann modulation contrast or differential interference contrast (DIC) and 10x, 20x and 40x objectives
- Two micromanipulators (one for moving the holding pipette and another for moving the injection pipette holder)
- Adapter for inverted microscope
- Air holding pipette for the oocyte and injection pipette for transferring the sperm.

Consumables and Media

- Light mineral oil
- Shallow Petri dishes, tissue-culture-grade (e.g. 351006 Petri dishes (BD Falcon)) holding capillaries

- Transfer Tips (ICSI) injection capillaries
- Culture media (HEPES-buffered, supplemented with antibiotics, protein and pyruvate).

Microinjection Dish Preparation

It is essential to bring all media and oil to 37°C prior to use. For ICSI, place one droplet of PVP and several droplets of medium in the center of a Petri dish. Two larger droplets may also be needed for the storage of spermatozoa and/or equilibration of the capillaries. Then the droplets are completely covered with light mineral oil to maintain the stability of droplets as well as the temperature and osmolarity. Once prepared, the microinjection dish may be placed into the incubator until required.

Preparation of the Microinjection Capillaries

The microcapillaries have to be fitted, aligned and equilibrated before starting the ICSI procedure. Since the holding pipette is much bigger than the injection pipette, it can be used as a guide for positioning and equilibrating. First, the micropipettes have to be fitted into the universal capillary holder, which is connected to the microinjector via a tube. When working with oil-filled systems, please make sure that no air bubbles are in the system. Gently push the capillaries past the sealing rings inside the tool holder. After attaching the universal capillary holder, check the alignment. The injection angle can be adjusted independently.

To align the capillary in the vertical position, the universal capillary holder can be rotated, even when the pipette is tightly gripped in place. Both pipettes have to appear straight in the field of view.

The alignment in the horizontal plane has to be done with great care. The following points must be taken into account: the holding pipette has to be aligned without tilt, as it needs to lie flat on the bottom of the dish in order to aspirate the oocyte in a controlled manner. In contrast, the injection pipette needs to tilt downwards slightly so that the tail of the spermatozoon can be broken properly. It is also necessary to prime micropipettes with medium before use so that the manipulated gametes never come into contact with air or oil. Usually, equilibration is achieved using ICSI media.

Procedure of Microinjection

Load the sperms into the PVP drop. Place each oocyte into one of the medium drops. Press the joystick button twice to lower the injection needle (ICSI) capillary to position. At 200x magnification immobilize a sperm cell either by a quick movement of the ICSI capillary via the tail or by pressing the tail of the sperm cell against the bottom of the dish.

Aspirate the sperm cell, tail-first, into the ICSI capillary as flatly as possible by rotating the knob of the injector. Press the joystick button twice to move the transfer capillary which now contains the sperm cell up into the overlay medium. Move the Petri dish until you can see an oocyte in one of the surrounding drops and bring it into focus. Move the holding capillary to the oocyte droplet. The oocyte is attached gently but firmly to the holding capillary with the help of negative pressure created by the Air device. The first polar body should be in the

6-o-clock or 12-o-clock position; therefore you may need to turn the oocyte with the help of the ICSI capillary which has been lowered again to oocyte droplet until the polar body comes to rest in either position.

Then sharply focus on the ICSI injection needle and the oocyte, move the spermatozoon along the capillary and bring it to rest at its very tip by rotating the knob of the injector. By moving the joystick slightly, carefully push the transfer capillary through the zona pellucida and the oolemma into the ooplasm at 3-o-clock. The oocyte should be pricked in the middle so that the oolema membrane is gently and atraumatically broken. Advance the injection pipette and aspirate to the ooplasma into the injection capillary to be sure that the membrane is ruptured. Deposit the aspirated ooplasm and the spermatozoon towards the center of the oocyte. To introduce a minimal volume of the medium and PVP solution into the cytoplasm, gently withdraw the transfer capillary after the head of the sperm cell has left the pipette tip. Release the injected oocyte from the holding capillary and move both capillaries to position 2 by pressing the joystick button twice. If several oocytes are obtained, only three to four oocytes are injected as a rule. They are placed into cleavage medium and the remaining oocytes are then injected.

Assessment of Fertilization

About 16 to 18 hours after microinjection, check the oocytes for the presence of pronuclei and polar bodies. After another 24 hours, score the embryos (e.g. equal size of blastomeres) and transfer them into the uterus.

INTRACYTOPLASMIC MORPHOLOGICALLY SELECTED SPERM INJECTION (IMSI)

A sophisticated advancement to ICSI is IMSI, intracytoplasmic morphologically selected sperm injection, a method described by Bartoov et al. Prior to sperm injection, the morphology of the sperm cell is evaluated with high magnification DIC microscopy. Preceding studies have already demonstrated the advantage of IMSI over the conventional IVF-ICSI procedure in terms of the pregnancy rate.

PETRI DISH ICSI (PICSI)

Mature spermatozoa may selectively bind to hyaluronic acid. Diminished sperm maturity (failure of spermatogenetic membrane remodeling) may be related to increased levels of chromosomal aberrations. Solid-state HA binding would facilitate the selection of individual mature sperm with low levels of chromosomal aneuploidies. A drop of washed spermatozoa is placed close to the edge of the HA spot (in the special Petri dish).

Spermatozoa are allowed to migrate spontaneously. HA-bounded spermatozoa are collected with the ICSI micropipette.

BIBLIOGRAPHY

1. Alex C Varghese, Peter Bjoblom, Jayaprakashan (Eds). A practical guide to setting up an IVF lab and embryo culture systems. Jaypee Brothers Medical Publishers (In press).
2. Peter Nagy, Alex C Varghese, Ashok Agarwal (Eds). Practical manual of *in vitro* fertilization: Newer methods and novel devices, Springer-Verlag, USA (In press).
3. Varghese AC, Amir Arsalan and Agarwal A. An update on developments and future prospects of ICSI. Arch Med Sci. 2009;5(1A): S109-14.
4. Varghese AC, Goldberg E and Agarwal A. Current and future perspectives on intracytoplasmic sperm injection (ICSI): A critical commentary Reproductive Biomedicine Online. 2007;15, 6, 719-27.

14

Juan G Alvarez

IMSI and PICSI Sperm Selection

IMSI PROTOCOL

1. Place on the left side of the petri dish three observation 4 μL droplets made up of polyvinylpyrrolidone medium at decreasing concentrations (undiluted, 3% and 0%).
2. In the middle, place a 4 μL droplet (selection droplet) in HEPES/Ham's F-10 medium supplemented with 20% serum substitute supplement to store the selected spermatozoa.
3. On the right side, place one to three 4 μL droplets (injection droplets) in HEPES/Ham's F-10 medium supplemented with 20% serum supplement to host the oocytes to be microinjected by the ICSI procedure herein described.
4. Place all microdroplets under sterile liquid paraffin.
5. Place aliquots of the processed spermatozoa into the observation droplets for IMSI selection by means of either an inverted microscope equipped with Nomarski differential interference contrast optics or using the Leyca system. Capture images with a DXC-990P color video camera (x6600 magnification) and visualized on the monitor screen.
6. Spermatozoa with severe malformations, such as a pin, amorphous, tapered, round or multinucleated head, which can be identified clearly even by low magnification (x200 to x400), were not considered for IMSI selection.
7. In order to perform the sperm selection adequately, the embryologists have to follow each apparently suitable single sperm cell by moving the microscopic stage in the x, y and z directions until they observe even the smallest details. Spermatozoa with abnormal head size were excluded.
8. Only motile spermatozoa with normal head dimensions, and with no or a maximum of one vacuole (0.78 ± 0.18 μm) are retrieved from the observation droplets and aspirated into a sterilized glass non-angulated pipette with a 9 μm inner diameter tip (Humagen, Charlottesville, VA, USA). Spermatozoa are then placed into the selection droplet and finally used for injection into the oocytes by conventional ICSI (Palermo *et al.* 1992).
9. The selection normal spermatozoa according to the IMSI criteria may take between of 1 hour and 3 hour, depending on the quality of the semen sample.

PICSI PROTOCOL

1. Add the sperm to the pre-hydrated microdot in a volume equal to or greater than that used to prehydrate the dot (approximately 10 μL).
2. Touch the tip of the micropipette containing the sperm to the edge of the hydrating drop at the bottom of the dish under the oil and expel the sperm. By delivering the sperm in a volume equal to the hydrating fluid, immediate mixing and delivery of sperm to the vicinity of the microdot is assured. If the sperm are delivered in a smaller volume at the edge of the drop, a long time (> 30 min) may be required for them to swim through the hydrating fluid to the vicinity of the microdot. Once bound, hyaluronan-bound sperm are easily identified: they exhibit no progressive migration despite a vigorous tail cross-beat frequency.
3. To rapidly populate the microdot with bound sperm, approximately 100,000 hyaluronan-binding sperm per mL (approximately 1,000–2,000 total sperm in 10–20 μL volume) are needed over the microdot. As time passes, the number of bound sperm will increase as more swimming sperm make contact with the hyaluronan microdot.
4. Select sperm from the interior of the microdot. The wall of the hyaluronan microdot is a physical barrier to which many sperm will bind since this is usually the first point of contact. It is sometimes difficult to distinguish whether the sperm are bound or they are simply swimming against the edge of the microdot. If the density of bound sperm is too high or too low for good sperm selection, dilute or concentrate the prepared sperm sample and use the adjusted sperm sample to seed the next microdot.
5. To collect bound sperm, position the tip of the ICSI micropipette next to the sperm and gently suck fluid into the pipette, drawing in the sperm. Continue collecting until 20 to 50 sperm are captured. Expel the captured sperm into a PVP drop to process them for ICSI (inactivating the tail, re-evaluating motility and morphology). From the PVP droplet, select and load single, processed sperm for injection into the oocytes according to your standard injection protocol.
6. Sperm bind best to hyaluronan hydrogel at temperatures below 30°C. At temperatures above 30°C, sperm swimming vigor increases and the swimming force may overcome the binding force. The result is that about one-third of sperm bound at room temperature will show some progressive migration at 37°C and may be deemed not bound, e.g. immature. In practice, most ICSI microscope stages are heated to 37°C. PICSI dishes placed on a 37°C heated stage will come to about 33°C and then remain at that temperature. At 33°C or even at 37°C, many bound sperm will still be available for selection.

Juan G Alvarez

15 Oocyte Spindle Imaging System

INTRODUCTION

Quantitative birefringence imaging studies are performed with the Oosight™ from CRi (Woburn, MA). This instrument consists of a liquid-crystal tunable filter optic, a circular polarizer/green interference filter optic (these are compatible with most research-grade microscopes), a scientific-grade CCD camera and software for image acquisition and analysis. The system merges polarized light imaging with the precision of single-point analysis by accurately and precisely quantifying the magnitude and orientation of birefringence at every pixel in the field of view in near real-time.

Especifically, it is the quantitative nature of the images produced that elevates the technique above a mere contrast mechanism and enables machine vision identification and classification of morphological structures. These quantitative measurements provide the reproducible indices needed for rating developmental potential.

The meiotic spindle is an effective marker of oocyte viability. This dynamic organelle plays a pivotal role in ensuring normal fertilization and development. The absence of a birefringent spindle has been linked to poor fertilization and developmental potential. Data from multiple studies has established that approximately 10% of oocytes about to undergo ICSI lack a visible spindle, and embryos (Rienzi 2003, Wang 2001, Konc 2004). The absence of a spindle may be due to a variety of factors, including biological disruption or timing. Side-by-side imaging with confocal systems has demonstrated that some oocytes lacking a birefringent spindle also showed disrupted tubulin. In addition, recent data gathered with birefringence imaging support the idea that some oocytes may not yet be fully mature, even though they have an extruded polar body (Cohen 2004, Montag 2006). These oocytes may need more time to develop. The absence of a spindle can also be due to environmental factors, indicating suboptimal clinical procedures or conditions (Keefe 1999, Wang 2001). Therefore, environmental conditions should be scrutinized when any laboratory is generating oocytes with no birefringent spindles in the majority of the population, noting that the population should consist of multiple patients across multiple age groups and backgrounds.

Further analysis of spindles reveals that, if they are present, their amount of birefringence is indicative of their integrity. A spindle that is not fully intact or misshapen will have a lower birefringence than normal. Fluorescence microscopy has demonstrated that chromosomal displacement is highly correlated to spindle irregularity. Battaglia et al (1996) demonstrated that both chromosome displacement and spindle irregularity increase with advancing maternal age. A study by Liu et al. (2002) described diminished birefringence and abnormally shaped spindles in senescence-aged mouse oocytes, thereby showing that birefringence data is related to age-related spindle abnormalities in the mouse. In a reproductive toxicology study, mammalian oocytes that had been treated with a microtubule inhibitor had decreased birefringence and decreased spindle length in relation to the control group, correlating birefringence measurements with the amount of tubulin (Shen, 2005). Spindle imaging has also been applied to monitoring the health of oocytes before and after vitrification (Chen, 2004). Thus, when accurate numerical data can be gathered to characterize spindles, more subtle indicators of oocyte viability can be made available to embryologists.

Another metric that may be derived, once the spindle has been visualized, relates to its location. The spindle is a key organelle in the creation of the polar body and ought to remain near to it thereafter. A polar body that has moved far from the spindle may have been dislocated by some trauma. Studies have shown that spindles that are more than 90 degrees distant from the polar body correlate with poor embryo viability (Rienzi, 2003).

Spindle location can be used as more than just a metric: it can also guide the ICSI process itself. It is common to use the polar body as a landmark to orient an oocyte prior to ICSI so that the sperm is injected at a site compatible with correct cleavage orientation. However, research has shown that the spindle is a better marker of the true animal pole (Cooke, 2003). Cooke et al. found that embryos from spindle-aligned oocytes at the time of ICSI had an increase in all measured development parameters over control siblings.

In addition to the spindle, birefringence imaging can be used to view the layers of the zona pellucida. Zona organization plays a vital role in normal fertilization and development. Birefringence imaging can be used to assess the density, orientation and thickness of the zona, which has been shown to be a meaningful indicator of oocyte status (Shen 2005, Pelletier 2004).

OOSIGHT IMAGING PROTOCOL

1. After oocyte retrieval, oocytes should be matured *in vitro.*
2. Following *in vitro* maturation, the oocytes should be denuded using the standard hyaluronidase protocol before they can be placed on the oosight instrumentation for spindle visualization.
3. Spindle analysis should be performed at 37ºC on either fresh or cryopreserved oocytes.

Several other features of the oocyte can be visualized by birefringence imaging, including vacuoles (image), the oolemma and cytoskeletal fragments in the cytoplasm. These features have been less well studied than the spindle and the zona, but may hold further information of interest to clinicians.

The different imaging tools available to embryologists must be thought of as components in a kit; no single modality offers everything. Birefringence imaging, too, has limitations. One such is the necessity to manipulate the spindle into the plane of focus in order to obtain correct data. Another is the need to standardize procedures if reproducibility is to be attained. Yet a third is the inability of birefringence imaging to reveal the sperm or any special characteristics thereof. However, despite these limitations, this new modality succeeds in providing useful new information to embryologists.

BIBLIOGRAPHY

1. Bolton VN, Hawes SM, Taylor CT, Parsons JH. Development of spare human preimplantation embryos *in vitro:* An analysis of the correlations among gross morphology, cleavage rates, and development to the blastocyst. J IVF-ET. 1989;6(1):30-5.
2. Chen JC, Warshaw JB, Sanadi DR. Regulation of mitochondrial respiration in senescence. J Cell Phys. 1972;80:141-8.
3. Chen CK, Wang CW, Tsai Wj, Hsieh LL, Wang HS, Soong YK. Evaluation of meiotic spindles in thawed oocytes after vitrification using polarized light microscopy. Fertil Steril. 2004;82:666-72.
4. Cooke S, Tyler JP, Driscoll GL. Meiotic spindle location and identification and its effect on embryonic cleavage plane and early development. Hum Reprod. 2003;18:2397-2405.
5. Cohen M Malcov, Schwartz T, Mey-Raz N, Carmon A, Cohen T, Lessing JB, Amit A, Azem F. Spindle imaging: A new marker for optimal timing of ICSI? Hum Reprod. 2004;19(3):649.
6. Cory P, Keefe DL, Trimarchi JR. Noninvasive polarized light microscopy qunatitatively distinguishes the multilaminar structure of the zona pellicida of living human oocytes and embryos. Fert Steril. 2004;81:850-6.
7. Fleming JE, Miquel J, Cottrell SF, et al. Is cell aging caused by respiration-dependent injury to the mitochondrial genome? Gerontology. 1982;28:44-53.
8. Harman D. The biologic clock: The mitochondria? J Am Geri Soc. 1972;4:145-7.
9. Konc J, Kanyo K and Cseh S. Visualization and examination of the meiotic spindle in human oocytes with PolScope J Assist Reprod Genet. 2004;21:349-53.
10. Miquel J, Economos AC, Fleming J, Johnson Jr. JE. Mitochondrial role in aging. Exp Geront. 1980;15:575-91.
11. Moon JH, Hyun CS, Lee SW, Son WY, Yoon SH, Lim JH. Visualization of the metaphase II meiotic spindle in living human oocytes using the PolScope enables the prediction of embryonic developmental competence after ICSI. Hum Reprod. 2003;18(4):817-20.
12. Nohl H. Oxygen radical release in mitochondria: Influence of age. Free Radicals, Aging, and Degenerative Diseases. 1986.pp.77-97.
13. Richter C. Do mitochondrial DNA fragments promote cancer and aging? FEBS Letters. 1988; 241(1):1-5.
14. Riley JCM, Behrman HR. Oxygen radicals and reactive oxygen species in reproduction. PSEBM. 1991;198:781-91.
15. Shen Y, Stalf T, Mehnert C, Eichenlaub-Riter U, Tinneberg HR. High magnitude of light retardation by the zona pellucida is associated with conception cycles. Hum Reprod. 2005;20:1596-606.
16. Rienzi L, Ubaldi F, Martinez F, Iacobelli M, Minasi MG, Ferrero S, Tesarik J, Greco E. Relationship between meiotic spindle location with regard to the polar body position and oocyte developmental potential after ICSI. Hum Reprod. 2003;18(6):1289-93.
17. Wang WH, Meng L, Hackett RJ, Keefe DL. Developmental ability of human oocytes with or without birefringent spindles imaged by Polscope before insemination. Hum Reprod. 2001;16(7):1464-8.
18. Weimer KE, Hoffman DI, Maxson WS, et al. Embryonic morphology and rate of implantation of human embryos following co-culture on bovine oviductal epithelial cells. Hum Reprod. 1993;8(1):97-101.

16 Semen Cryopreservation and Banking

Pankaj Talwar

INTRODUCTION

The banking of the male gametes involves initial exposure of the spermatozoa to the cryoprotectant and gradually cooling them to subzero temperatures as per desired cooling curve.[1] Semen sample in suitable container is then cryopreserved in liquid nitrogen at –196° centigrade till required. When required Cryobioreposited semen sample is then thawed, gradually warmed to the room temperature and diluted with suitable buffered media. Cryoprotectant is washed away and the thawed sample evaluated and used for insemination, Intra Cytoplasmic Sperm Injection or for research purposes.

The male gamete must maintain its macro and micro architectural structure along with genomic integrity during the whole procedure and recover its physiological functions completely after the procedure.[2]

Factors known to effect outcome of this delicate procedure depends upon the quality of the semen specimen, developmental stage at which sperms are being frozen, type of cryoprotectant being used and the freezing protocols.[3]

INDICATIONS OF SEMEN CRYOPRESERVATION

Sperm banking is the process of semen cryopreservation using well documented protocols for use of the same at a later date. Semen can be preserved for the use by the individual himself.[4] The sample can be used by him at a later date and is termed as autologous sperm banking or client depositor semen cryofreezing.[5] It can be also banked from fertile donors after screening for the purpose of third party reproduction (Table 16.1).

Adequate care is taken to do phenotypic/blood group matching in these cases. Matching physical characteristics and race of the partner, hair color, texture and eye color are mandatory. The indications of semen banking are ever increasing in this modern era. The common indications are enumerated in Table 16.2.

OUTLINE OF CRYOPROTECTANTS

All the cryopreservation protocol are based on the theory that cell membrane damage can be minimized through addition of suitable cryoprotective agents, buffer agents, controlling the

Table 16.1: Terminologies used in semen banking

Terminologies	*Description*
Cryopreservation	The sub-branch of cryobiology that deals with the reversible suspension of life in the frozen state at subzero temperatures using cryoprotectants
Quarantine	Temporary storage/isolation of semen in a separate cryocans till the donor is proved negative for the communicable disease agent
Sperm Bank	A facility that collects, freezes, stores and distributes semen sample
Client Depositor	Patient who cryopreserved his semen for insemination of a partner at latter date
Donor	One who provides his own semen for cryobanking for artificial insemination of a recipient other than his wife or partner
Directed Donor	A sperm donor who may know the recipient and directs the laboratory to freeze his semen for use by specific individuals who are not his partner
Anonymous Donor	A semen donor whose identity is not revealed to the recipient

Table 16.2: Current approaches to semen banking

Clinical presentation of the male requiring semen banking	Method of sperm harvesting	Method of semen banking
Male with normal /or low semen count and desires autologous semen banking	Semen obtained by masturbation/ electro-ejaculation	Raw/prepared semen freezing
Azoospermic males in reproductive age group		
Obstructive (LH, FSH within normal limits)	Sample extracted from the epididymis: Percutaneous epididymal sperm aspiration (PESA)	Freezing of the epididymal aspirate either unprepared or after gentle wash and swim-up
Nonobstructive (FSH may be raised)	MESA: Microsurgical epididymal sperm aspiration TESE: Testicular epididymal sperm extraction	Freezing of the testicular tissue is done after gentle teasing in a sterile dish using fine needles
	TESA: Testicular epididymal sperm aspiration	Tissue is frozen either unprepared or after density gradient wash
Cancer patients prior chemotherapy or radiotherapy		
Prepubertal boys	Testicular tissue (multiple samples)	Freezing of the testicular tissue
Pubertal	Masturbation	Semen banking

Table 16.3: Types of cryoprotectants

	Mechanism of action	*Names*
Permeating	Permeating cryoprotectants are compounds that readily permeate the plasma membranes of cells Their movements across the membranes follow the osmolarity gradient These molecules form hydrogen bonds with water molecules and prevent ice crystallization	Dimethylsulfoxide (DMSO), propylene glycol, glycerol Glycerol is commonly used for semen freezing
Nonpermeating	Nonpermeating cryoprotectants are large molecules that remain extracellular These create osmolarity gradient by drawing water from within the cell, thus dehydrating the intracellular space Can be toxic to the cells at higher temperatures and after prolonged exposure Used in combination with the permeating cryoprotectants to prevent cytotoxicity	Sucrose, raffinose, and glycine

osmolality and pH of cryopreservation medium and controlling the freezing rate during the procedure.[6]

A variety of extenders (Cryoprotective Media) exist for the cooling and cryopreservation of semen (Table 16.3). The purpose of the extender is manifold. The media contains nutrient, a buffer, a cryoprotectant agent and antibiotic. A typical nutrient added is a sugar, such as glucose or sucrose, which serves to provide energy source for the sperm. Buffers are added to balance pH and osmolarity of the solution. An ideal biological buffer should have a pH value between 6 and 8.[7] The role of the buffer in cryopreservation is to pickup hydrogen ions in the surrounding media, thereby assisting in dehydration of the cell and maintaining a neutral pH.

ESSENTIALS OF FREEZE-THAW CYCLE

Decision of semen packaging protocol before the procedure and it's importance to the reproductive biologist

Semen parameters should be thoroughly assessed using WHO criterion. We should decide the outcome of the procedure which will further guide the freezing protocol. If the sample is satisfactory with good count and motility, we may freeze raw sample with aim to carry out IUI at latter date. On the other hand, an oligospermic sample with round cells and debris should be prepared and packaged for ICSI. Finally, the methodology depends upon the experience of the reproductive biologist and the laboratory protocols.

Specimen glycerolization

Glycerol is added directly or indirectly, as a component of a Cryopreservation medium, to neat semen /prepared semen (swim-up) in drop by drop fashion slowly over a period of 2 to

Table 16.4: Guidelines for better recovery

	Preventive strategies	*Guidelines*
1.	Freezing initiation	To avoid cytotoxic effects (reactive oxygen species) release from immotile/dead spermatozoa, it is suggested that the semen sample is prepared and frozen soon after collection. Raw sample may also be banked but immediately after liquefaction.
2.	Accidental thawing	The sperm plasma membrane is very sensitive. Careless handling of the frozen semen straw will injure the spermatozoal plasma and acrosomal membranes resulting in a low sperm survival rate after thawing.
3.	Cryoprotectant removal after thawing	Glycerol as a cryoprotectant is toxic for sperms if exposed for long period at room or higher temperatures.Thus post-thaw survival should quickly be assessed and the sperm sample washed to remove all traces of glycerol.

3 minutes, with continuous mixing of both. This step is essential to reduce toxicity of the cryoprotectant as it can cause sudden osmotic shock to the sperms. The glycerol is metabolized during the procedure with formation of neutral lipid. It is suggested that the metabolized glycerol may contribute to the plasma membrane of the sperm increasing its stability which may lead to improved post-thaw motility[8] (Table 16.4).

Packaging of semen after addition of cryopreservative

Glycerated or extended semen can be cryopreserved in various containers. Factors, which influence the decisions, include the volume of sample to be cryopreserved, ease of container labeling, handling, storage, and recovery as well as biocompatibility of the packaging material (Table 16.5).

Cooling and warming rates

The outcome of sperm cryosurvival is related to the rate at which the cells are cooled and warmed.[9]

Freezing (Table 16.6)

Sperm cryopreservation is accomplished using liquid nitrogen vapors for noncontrolled rate or a programmable freezer for controlled rate cooling. Regardless of the cooling process, the ultimate quality control appraisal of sperm cryopreservation is the cryosurvival of the spermatozoa determined during thawing.[10]

Storage

Once specimens attain temperature of –80°C to –120 °C, they are immediately plunged into liquid nitrogen. After plunging, the vials are quickly transferred to a precooled, labeled aluminum can/goblet for storage in liquid phase of liquid nitrogen tank .When freezing semen by non-controlled rate protocol, vials may be loaded onto the aluminum cane prior to cryopreservation to eliminate the need for transfer after cryopreservation. Every effort should be made to limit the time; specimens spend out of the liquid phase of liquid nitrogen.

Table 16.5: Packaging of the semen sample

		Advantages	*Disadvantages*
Straws	Ionomeric resin CBS High Security (CryoBioSystem, Paris,France)	Straws are available in a variety of colors suitable for the easy identification of samples, and many hundred's can be stored in plastic goblets in canisters within liquid nitrogen containers	1. Maximum capacity of approximately 0.5 mL only 2. Overfilled straws are prone to cracking and expelling the powder sealing plugs into the liquid nitrogen 3. Labeling and filling difficulties 4. A high surface/ volume ratio which makes the sample very susceptible to warming shock damage resulting from exposure to ambient temperatures during handling
Cryovials	Polypropylene with screw caps	These are easy to fill and stores nearly 1.5 mL of the of semen plus cryoprotectant mixture	1. Storage on aluminum canes is not dependable as they lose their memory and cryovials may jump off the holder 2. Screw-top vials do not maintain their seals. They have the potential of exploding upon thawing because liquid nitrogen trapped in the vials expand to many times its volume when it converts to gaseous nitrogen 3. The low surface: Volume ratio and thick wall of the cryovial increase the time required for samples to reach critical temperatures and thus increase the risk of damage from brief exposure to ambient temperatures
Glass vials	Glass	None over the other available cryocon-tainers	Glass vials are very fragile thus there use is discouraged

Straws are quickly transferred to precooled, labeled plastic goblets, snapped onto a labeled aluminum can. Straws should be oriented in the goblet so that identifying information can be read without completely withdrawing the straw from the goblet. Aluminum cans are placed in predetermined locations within the cryostorage vessel. All storage containers should be stored in a secured room in locked /chained containers. Liquid nitrogen dewars and storage tanks are available in a variety of sizes. Dewars require manual filling while most storage tanks have an automatic filling feature. Liquid nitrogen levels in storage units should be monitored regularly at all times. It is important to appreciate the length of time cryopreserved sperm may be stored for. At –196°C, storage of sperms, even for a lengthy period of time, does not affect the survival rates. Liquid nitrogen holds specimens at a temperature (–196°C) at which there is virtually no

Table 16.6: Sperm freezing step by step

	Sample preparation	
Sperm Cryopreservation Method	1. Ensure both the sample and sperm Cryopreservation buffer (K-SISC) are at room temperature 2. Mix two volumes of sperm Cryopreservation buffer to 1 volume of sample 3. Leave mixture for 10 minutes at room temperature 4. Label straws with relevant information 5. Load the sample into a freezing straw or cryovial and seal according to manufacturer's instructions **Freezing** A controlled rate freezing system is recommended for freezing using liquid nitrogen vapor, however results could vary such method should be validated by the individual laboratory	
Freezing	*Straws*	*Cryovials*
	Load straws into freezing machine and initiate freeze program for straws should have similar parameters to the given below: • Start temperature is 20°C • Cooling rate of 6°C/min until –80°C • At –80°C plunge them into liquid nitrogen	Load cryovials into freezing machine and initiate freeze program. The freeze program for cryovials should have similar parameters to those given below: • Start temperature is 20°C • Cooling rate of –0.5°C/ min to + 5.0°C • At + 5.0°C cool at a rate of –1°C/ min to +4.0°C • At + 4.0°C cool at rate of 2°C /min to + 3.0°C • At +3.0°C cool at a rate of –4°C /min to +2.0°C • At +1.0°C cool at a rate of –10°C /min to –80.0°C • At +80°C hold for 10 minutes • Plunge into liquid nitrogen
Thawing	1. Remove straws or cryovials from liquid nitrogen and place them at room temperature until thawing is complete 2. Open the straws or cryo-tube and remove the thawed semen 3. Dilute the semen with Gamete buffer (1:1) to reduce the toxic effect of glycerol 4. Quickly evaluate the survival of the sperm. Immediately prepare sperm by the density gradient method using Sperm gradient or the swim-up	

movement of atoms or molecules. At temperatures above –130°C, atoms, and molecules are able to move. Temperatures of –90°C and above allow ice crystal growth and even short periods of exposure to such temperatures can cause lethal damage to cells. As long as the cells are maintained at –196°C, the only known potential for cell damage is degradation of deoxyribonucleic acid (DNA) caused by background radiation. Based on normal background radiation of 0.1 rads/year, it has been predicted that the male gametes should maintain its genetic integrity for over 200 years when stored at –196°C.

Thawing

Practical approach to semen thawing would be to wash the vials /straws in running water. They should be cleaned externally till the sweating disappears over a period of few minutes. Once the sample is thawed, mix the sample well with a pipette before sampling. Perform the sperm count and assess the motility as per WHO guidelines. Specimen should be processed immediately after post-thaw analysis.

LEGISLATION PERTAINING TO THE SEMEN BANKING

Indian Council of Medical Research has issued comprehensive guidelines for Assisted Reproductive Technologies centers. These are guidelines which may be applied to any functioning semen bank, an ART clinic or a law firm or any other suitable independent organization may set up a semen bank.

- All donors should produce their semen samples within the collection area of the center so that the sample cannot be substituted by others semen sample. It is essential that there is suitable privacy, time and environment for patients to do this.
- Donor records and coding of the specimens stored must be kept securely. The centers should audit their cryobanks annually.
- The semen bank shall not supply semen of one donor for more than ten successful pregnancies. It will be the responsibility of the ART clinic or the patient, to inform the bank about a successful pregnancy.
- The bank shall keep a record of all semen received, stored, and supplied, and details of the use of the semen of each donor. This record will be liable to be reviewed by the accreditation authority.
- A semen bank may store a semen preparation for exclusive use on the donor's wife or on any other woman designated by the donor.
- An appropriate charge may be levied by the bank for the storage. In the case of non-payment of the charges when the donor is alive, the bank would have the right to destroy the semen sample or give it to a bonafide organization to be used only for research purposes. In the case of the death of the donor, the semen would become the property of the legal heir or the nominee of the donor at the time the donor gives the sample for storage to the bank.
- In the United Kingdom, the semen is not normally stored for longer than 10 years or beyond the age of 55 years for donors; generally it is not stored in France for more than 5 years.
- Donors may express a wish to further limit the period of storage or the number of pregnancies that can be obtained from one donor. This is restricted to 10 children by the same donor. Confidentiality remains a primary consideration in most countries.

DONOR SCREENING PRIOR TO SEMEN BANKING

- Fresh donor insemination is not recommended for the fear of transmission of common infective diseases.
- Donors should be tested for HIV 1 and 2, HTLV I and II antibodies, hepatitis B surface antigen, hepatitis B core antibody, hepatitis C, RPR, TP-PA , cytomegalovirus antibodies,

chlamydia and gonorrhea. Some agents and diseases that can be transmitted by the seminal fluid include HIV, hepatitis B, hepatitis C and syphilis.

- Donors are screened for the infections at the time of presentation.
- As a donor may be in window period of an infection, it is necessary to repeat the examination for hepatitis B and HIV after an appropriate quarantine period of 180 days.
- If the history or physical examination indicates infection, the donor should be rejected and advised to seek appropriate medical advise.
- Donor should be thoroughly screened for common genetic and communicable diseases and those specific to their geographic location before their enrolment in the program.

CROSSINFECTION IN THE SEMEN BANKS

There is a potential danger of cross-infection within the bank thus the samples must be handled and stored with paramount care.

- Cryopreserved semen may be spilled in the cryocan, and the infectious organism (hepatitis B virus) may survive in the liquid nitrogen with the possibility of cross-infection of other stored samples.
- It is recommended that samples be stored in isolation cryocans till the quarantine period of HIV, HbsAg and HCV.
- Use of CBS ionomeric straws which have been hermetically sealed offers protection against cross infection.
- Men with malignancy often need to bank their semen at short notice as to preclude complete pre freeze infective screening. These men's semen could be reposited in a quarantine tank until the requisite screening had been completed.
- Client depositor/autologous who has the comfort of time, e.g. men considering a vasectomy, a cryobank must insist upon screening for infective pathogens as a safety precaution for the security of other men's semen stored in the same canister.
- When the samples are cryopreserved for patients who are known to carry an infective infection, e.g. HIV/HBsAg. These can be stored in separate 'contaminated' tanks.
- There must be a separate tank for each of recognized pathogenic organisms. In the United States and United Kingdom, guidelines have been published. The HEFA is moving toward a position whereby laboratories will be compelled to screen donors in this way.

SECURITY OF THE SEMEN BANK

- The straws or vials must be clearly labeled.
- Inventory control is of utmost importance. Every precaution must be made to ensure that each straw or vial can be linked to the sperm source, date of cryopreservation and specimen number, canister/cane or rack/cryocan number.
- The cryocans have a locking facility which must be utilized and limited staff allowed access to the keys. Some example of vial or straw identification mechanisms currently employed by sperm banks include: Computerized or manual bar coding system, color coding with cryomarkers, vial caps or straw plugs or use of adhesive labels.
- Secure cryopreservation of semen requires regular maintenance of the equipment and refilling of liquid nitrogen in the cryocans.

- Liquid nitrogen evaporates very quickly or the cans can leak thus causing loss of precious samples. The loss of stored semen from cancer or other patients like those having spinal cord injuries and in whom semen has been retrieved with electro-ejaculation is not only difficult to quantify but is of immense emotional value to the owner /couple.
- All the details and records must be stored confidentially and country specific guidelines adhered to when carrying out cryofreezing at the center.
- The following measures are considered customary by various accreditation authorities:
  - i. The levels of LN_2 in cryocans that are filled manually should be monitored on a regular basis, using a cryoscale.
  - ii. In large cryobiorepository cans may be attached to automated cryo manifold with 'auto-fill' controller.
  - iii. Low-level and temperature sensors should be installed in all cryogenic storage tanks and connected to an alarm that will alert biologist to unwarranted problems.

REFERENCES

1. Parkes AS. Preservation of human spermatozoa at low temperatures. Brit MJ. 1945;2:212-3.
2. Sherman JK, Buge RG. Observations on preservation of human spermatozoa at low temperatures. Proc Soc Exp Biol Med. 1953;82:686-8.
3. Hammerstedt RH, Graham JK, Nolan JP. Cryopreservation of mammalian sperm; what we ask them to survive. J Androl. 1990;11:73-88.
4. Shapiro SS. Strategies to improve efficiency of therapeutic donor insemination. In: Diamond MP, DeCherney AH, eds. Infertility and Reproductive Medicine Clinics in North America. Male infertility, Philadelphia: WB Saunders. 1992.pp.469-85.
5. Bordson BL, Ricci E, Dicky RP, Dunway H, Taylor SN, Curole DW. Comparison of fecundability with fresh and frozen semen in therapeutic donor insemation. Fertile Steril. 1986.pp.466-9.
6. Van den Berg L, Soliman FS. Composition and pH changes during freezing of solutions containing calcium and magnesium phosphate. Cryobiology. 1969;6:10-4.
7. Mortimer D. Semen Cryopreservation. In: Practical Laboratory Andrology. Oxford: Oxford University Press, 1994.
8. Mazur P. Freezing of living cells: mechanisms and implications. Am J Physiol. 1974;247:C125-42.
9. Tyler JPP, Kime L, Cooke S, Driscoll GL, Temperature change in cryo-containers during short exposure to ambient temperatures. Hum Reprod. 1996;11:1510-2.
10. Graham EF, Crabo BG. Some methods of freezing and evaluating human spermatozoa. Proc Natl Acad Sci. 1978;4:274-304.

17

Juan G Alvarez

Semen Vitrification

- Load 1 mL aliquot of the semen sample onto a 40/80 SpermFilter (Cryos International, Denmark) (or equivalent) density gradient.
- Centrifuge at 1600 rpm during 20 minutes.
- Aspirate pellet and resuspend in 2 mL of HTF medium (or equivalent) supplemented with 1% BSA.
- Centrifuge at 1800 rpm during 10 minutes.
- Resuspend pellet in a volume of HTF medium to obtain a maximal sperm concentration of 100 million spermatozoa/mL.
- Mix the resupended pellet with 0.5 M sucrose (1:1, v/v) to obtain a maximal final sperm concentration of 50 million/mL.
- Load 100 μL aliquots of the mixture into capillaries open at both ends (maximal count of 5 million spermatozoa per capillary).
- Insert capillary into CBS straw and thermo seal both ends.
- Immerse straw into liquid nitrogen for 1 second.
- Immediately transfer straw to the canister of liquid nitrogen cryogenic tank.
- For thawing, cut both ends of the straw and place capillary into a test tube containing 10 mL of HTF medium prewarmed at 37°C and supplemented with 1% BSA.
- Incubate capillary in prewarmed HTF medium for 5 minutes.
- Centrifuge at 1800 rpm during 5 minutes, discard supernatant and resuspend sperm pellet in the desired medium.
- Assess motility using a conventional light microscope. Motility recoveries using this vitrificacion protocol, usually range between 75 and 90%.

Index